Population Health in Rural America in 2020

PROCEEDINGS OF A WORKSHOP

Anna Nicholson, *Rapporteur*

Roundtable on Population Health Improvement

Board on Population Health and Public Health Practice

Health and Medicine Division

The National Academies of
SCIENCES · ENGINEERING · MEDICINE

THE NATIONAL ACADEMIES PRESS
Washington, DC
www.nap.edu

THE NATIONAL ACADEMIES PRESS   500 Fifth Street, NW   Washington, DC 20001

This activity was supported by contracts between the National Academy of Sciences and Aetna Foundation, Association of American Medical Colleges, Blue Shield of California Foundation, BlueCross BlueShield of North Carolina, The California Endowment, Fannie E. Rippel Foundation/ReThink Health, Geisinger, The Kresge Foundation, National Association of County and City Health Officials, Nemours, New York State Health Foundation, Robert Wood Johnson Foundation, Samueli Foundation, The University of Texas at Austin, Thomas Jefferson University, and Wake Forest Baptist Medical Center. Any opinions, findings, conclusions, or recommendations expressed in this publication do not necessarily reflect the views of any organization or agency that provided support for the project.

International Standard Book Number-13: 978-0-309-68527-6
International Standard Book Number-10: 0-309-68527-3
Digital Object Identifier: https://doi.org/10.17226/25989

Additional copies of this publication are available from the National Academies Press, 500 Fifth Street, NW, Keck 360, Washington, DC 20001; (800) 624-6242 or (202) 334-3313; http://www.nap.edu.

Copyright 2021 by the National Academy of Sciences. All rights reserved.

Printed in the United States of America

Suggested citation: National Academies of Sciences, Engineering, and Medicine. 2021. *Population health in rural America in 2020: Proceedings of a workshop.* Washington, DC: The National Academies Press. https://doi.org/10.17226/25989.

The National Academies of
SCIENCES · ENGINEERING · MEDICINE

The **National Academy of Sciences** was established in 1863 by an Act of Congress, signed by President Lincoln, as a private, nongovernmental institution to advise the nation on issues related to science and technology. Members are elected by their peers for outstanding contributions to research. Dr. Marcia McNutt is president.

The **National Academy of Engineering** was established in 1964 under the charter of the National Academy of Sciences to bring the practices of engineering to advising the nation. Members are elected by their peers for extraordinary contributions to engineering. Dr. John L. Anderson is president.

The **National Academy of Medicine** (formerly the Institute of Medicine) was established in 1970 under the charter of the National Academy of Sciences to advise the nation on medical and health issues. Members are elected by their peers for distinguished contributions to medicine and health. Dr. Victor J. Dzau is president.

The three Academies work together as the **National Academies of Sciences, Engineering, and Medicine** to provide independent, objective analysis and advice to the nation and conduct other activities to solve complex problems and inform public policy decisions. The National Academies also encourage education and research, recognize outstanding contributions to knowledge, and increase public understanding in matters of science, engineering, and medicine.

Learn more about the National Academies of Sciences, Engineering, and Medicine at **www.nationalacademies.org**.

The National Academies of
SCIENCES · ENGINEERING · MEDICINE

Consensus Study Reports published by the National Academies of Sciences, Engineering, and Medicine document the evidence-based consensus on the study's statement of task by an authoring committee of experts. Reports typically include findings, conclusions, and recommendations based on information gathered by the committee and the committee's deliberations. Each report has been subjected to a rigorous and independent peer-review process, and it represents the position of the National Academies on the statement of task.

Proceedings published by the National Academies of Sciences, Engineering, and Medicine chronicle the presentations and discussions at a workshop, symposium, or other event convened by the National Academies. The statements and opinions contained in proceedings are those of the participants and are not endorsed by other participants, the planning committee, or the National Academies.

For information about other products and activities of the National Academies, please visit www.nationalacademies.org/about/whatwedo.

PLANNING COMMITTEE ON POPULATION HEALTH IN RURAL AMERICA IN 2020[1]

TOM MORRIS (*Chair*), Federal Office of Rural Health Policy, Health Resources and Services Administration
MICHAEL BIRD, Indian Health Council
ALVA FERDINAND, Southwest Rural Health Research Center, Texas A&M University
ALANA KNUDSON, Walsh Center for Rural Health Analysis, NORC at the University of Chicago
JOSÉ T. MONTERO, Center for State, Tribal, Local, and Territorial Support; Centers for Disease Control and Prevention
KAREN MURPHY, The Steele Institute for Health Innovation, Geisinger
LARS PETERSON, Rural & Underserved Health Research Center, University of Kentucky

---

[1] The National Academies of Sciences, Engineering, and Medicine's planning committees are solely responsible for organizing the workshop, identifying topics, and choosing speakers. The responsibility for the published Proceedings of a Workshop rests with the workshop rapporteur and the institution.

ROUNDTABLE ON POPULATION HEALTH IMPROVEMENT[1]

SANNE MAGNAN (*Co-Chair*), Senior Fellow, HealthPartners Institute
JOSHUA M. SHARFSTEIN (*Co-Chair*), Associate Dean for Public Health Practice and Training, Johns Hopkins Bloomberg School of Public Health
PHILIP M. ALBERTI, Senior Director, Health Equity Research and Policy, Association of American Medical Colleges
DAWN ALLEY, Chief Strategy Officer, Center for Medicare & Medicaid Innovation, Centers for Medicare & Medicaid Services
JOHN AUERBACH, Executive Director, Trust for America's Health
CATHY BAASE, Chair, Board of Directors, Michigan Health Improvement Alliance; Consultant for Health Strategy, The Dow Chemical Company
RAYMOND BAXTER, Trustee, Blue Shield of California Foundation
DEBBIE I. CHANG, President and Chief Executive Officer, Blue Shield of California Foundation
MARC N. GOUREVITCH, Professor and Chair, Department of Population Health, New York University Langone Health
GARTH GRAHAM, President, Aetna Foundation
MEG GUERIN-CALVERT, Senior Managing Director and President, Center for Healthcare, Economics and Policy, FTI Consulting
GARY R. GUNDERSON, Vice President, Faith Health, School of Divinity, Wake Forest University
DORA HUGHES, Associate Research Professor of Health Policy and Management, Milken Institute School of Public Health, The George Washington University
SHERI JOHNSON, Director, Population Health Institute; Acting Director, Robert Wood Johnson Foundation, Culture of Health Prize; Associate Professor, Department of Population Health Sciences, School of Medicine and Public Health, University of Wisconsin–Madison
WAYNE JONAS, Executive Director, Integrative Health Programs, H&S Ventures; Samueli Foundation
ROBERT M. KAPLAN, Professor, Center for Advanced Study in the Behavioral Sciences, Stanford University
MICHELLE LARKIN, Associate Vice President, Associate Chief of Staff, Robert Wood Johnson Foundation

---

[1] The National Academies of Sciences, Engineering, and Medicines planning committees are solely responsible for organizing the workshop, identifying topics, and choosing speakers. The responsibility for the published Proceedings of a Workshop rests with the workshop rapporteur and the institution.

MILTON LITTLE, President, United Way of Greater Atlanta
PHYLLIS D. MEADOWS, Senior Fellow, Health Program, The Kresge Foundation
BOBBY MILSTEIN, Director, ReThink Health
JOSÉ T. MONTERO, Director, Center for State, Tribal, Local, and Territorial Support; Deputy Director, Centers for Disease Control and Prevention
WILLIE (BILLY) H. OGLESBY, Interim Dean, Jefferson College of Population Health, Thomas Jefferson University
JASON PURNELL, Associate Professor, Director, Health Equity Works, Brown School, Washington University in Saint Louis
RAHUL RAJKUMAR, Senior Vice President and Chief Medical Officer, BlueCross and BlueShield of North Carolina
LOURDES J. RODRIGUEZ, Senior Program Officer, St. David's Foundation
PAMELA RUSSO, Senior Program Officer, Robert Wood Johnson Foundation
KOSALI SIMON, Herman B. Wells Endowed Professor, Associate Vice Provost for Health Sciences, Paul H. O'Neill School of Public and Environmental Affairs, Indiana University
HANH CAO YU, Chief Learning Officer, The California Endowment

Health and Medicine Division Staff

ALINA BACIU, Roundtable Director
CARLA ALVARADO, Program Officer (*through January 2021*)
HARIKA DYER, Senior Program Assistant
AYSHIA COLETRANE, Senior Program Assistant (*from October 2020*)
ROSE M. MARTINEZ, Senior Board Director, Board on Population Health and Public Health Practice

Consultant

ANNA NICHOLSON, Rapporteur

Reviewers

This Proceedings of a Workshop was reviewed in draft form by individuals chosen for their diverse perspectives and technical expertise. The purpose of this independent review is to provide candid and critical comments that will assist the National Academies of Sciences, Engineering, and Medicine in making each published proceedings as sound as possible and to ensure that it meets the institutional standards for quality, objectivity, evidence, and responsiveness to the charge. The review comments and draft manuscript remain confidential to protect the integrity of the process.

We thank the following individuals for their review of this proceedings:

HARTLEY CARMICHAEL FELD, University of Kentucky College of Nursing
DANIELLE LUCERO, University of Washington

Although the reviewers listed above provided many constructive comments and suggestions, they were not asked to endorse the content of the proceedings nor did they see the final draft before its release. The review of this proceedings was overseen by **MARTIN J. SEPULVEDA,** IBM Corporation. He was responsible for making certain that an independent examination of this proceedings was carried out in accordance with standards of the National Academies and that all review comments were carefully considered. Responsibility for the final content rests entirely with the rapporteur and the National Academies.

Contents

	ACRONYMS AND ABBREVIATIONS	xv
1	**INTRODUCTION**	1
	Workshop Objectives, 2	
	Organization of the Proceedings, 3	
2	**RURAL AMERICA IN CONTEXT**	5
	Rural Demographics and Social Determinants of Health, 5	
	Structural Urbanism in Rural America, 12	
	Discussion, 17	
3	**RURAL HEALTH VITAL SIGNS**	21
	Why Is Mortality Higher in Rural America?, 21	
	Tribal Health Perspective, 25	
	Rural Data Challenges in the Healthy People 2020 Initiative, 29	
	Rural Healthy People Initiative: Processes and Rural Health Indicators, 31	
	The Effect of Racial Disparities in Rural Areas, 35	
	Discussion, 39	
4	**RURAL HEALTH CARE IN ACTION**	45
	Rural Health Care Landscape, 45	
	Tribal Health and Health Care in Rural Settings, 49	
	Wraparound Services: Implications for Rural America, 53	

The Role of Community Health Workers in Addressing
   the Needs of Rural Americans, 57
Discussion, 63

5   **ASSESSMENT AND IMPLEMENTATION
    STRATEGIES FOR IMPROVING THE HEALTH
    OF RURAL POPULATIONS**   69
    Community Health Needs Assessment, 69
    Minnesota Integrated Behavioral Health Program to Support
       Population Health, 73
    Role of Rural Development Hubs and Policy in Connecting
       Rural Development, Health, and Opportunity, 77
    Innovations in Sustaining Rural Population Health, 83
    Discussion, 88

6   **RURAL HEALTH POLICY**   93
    Shifting Rural Health Policy and Practice Toward
       Value-Based Care, 93
    Engaging Health Care Providers to Confront Rural
       America's Health Care Crisis, 97
    Tribal Rural Health Policy, 102
    Congressional Response to COVID-19 for Rural America, 107
    Discussion, 112

APPENDIXES

A	Speaker and Planning Committee Member Biosketches	117
B	Workshop Agenda	131
C	References	135

Boxes, Figures, and Table

BOXES

1-1 Statement of Task, 2

3-1 Alaska Pacific University, 26

4-1 Community Health Workers' Reflections on Their Roles, 59

5-1 Community Health Needs Assessment Process, 71

6-1 Margaret Mary Health, 94

FIGURES

2-1 Rural counties with more than 20 percent of their populations aged 65 years or older, 2017, 7

2-2 Race and ethnicity in rural areas, 9

3-1 Diverging trends in age-adjusted mortality in metro versus nonmetro areas in the United States, 23

3-2 Chronic disease burden by race and ethnicity for diabetes, 34

4-1 Wraparound services to address social determinants of health, 54

5-1 Blueprint for action for improving community health through innovations in financing, 86

TABLE

3-1 Top Rural Health Priorities Identified by Rural Healthy People 2010 and Rural Healthy People 2020, 33

Acronyms and Abbreviations

ACO	accountable care organization
AHRQ	Agency for Healthcare Research and Quality
ATHS	Alaska Tribal Health System
BPC	Bipartisan Policy Center
CAH	critical access hospital
CARES	Coronavirus Aid, Relief, and Economic Security
CCCHC	Coal Country Community Health Center
CDC	Centers for Disease Control and Prevention
CDC WONDER	CDC Wide-ranging Online Data for Epidemiologic Research
CHNA	community health needs assessment
CHR	community health representative
CHW	community health worker
CMS	Centers for Medicare & Medicaid Services
COPD	chronic obstructive pulmonary disease
COVID-19	coronavirus disease 2019
ED	emergency department
EHR	electronic health record
FQHC	federally qualified health center

HHS	Department of Health and Human Services
HRSA	Health Resources and Services Administration
IBH	integrated behavioral health
ICU	intensive care unit
IHCIA	Indian Health Care Improvement Act
IHS	Indian Health Service
KFF	Kaiser Family Foundation
medevac	medical evacuation
metro	metropolitan
OMB	Office of Management and Budget
PPE	personal protective equipment
PPP	Paycheck Protection Program
RAP	recommendation adoption progress
SBA	Small Business Administration
SDOH	social determinants of health
SMC	Sakakawea Medical Center

1

Introduction

To explore issues related to population health in rural America, the public virtual workshop Population Health in Rural America in 2020 was convened on June 24–25, 2020, by the Roundtable on Population Health Improvement of the Board on Population Health and Public Health Practice of the National Academies of Sciences, Engineering, and Medicine. The workshop was planned by a workshop planning committee composed of rural health experts representing public health, health care, and tribal health.[1] Rural America is economically, socially, culturally, geographically, and demographically diverse. This multidimensional diversity presents complex challenges and unique opportunities related to delivering health care and improving health outcomes in rural communities.

In her welcoming remarks, Sanne Magnan, Roundtable on Population Health Improvement co-chair and senior fellow from the HealthPartners Institute, explained that since 2013 the Roundtable on Population Health Improvement has provided a trusted venue for leaders from the public and private sectors to meet and discuss the leverage points and opportunities for achieving better population health. The roundtable's vision is to help create a strong, healthy, and productive society that cultivates

---

[1] The planning committee's role was limited to planning the workshop, and the Proceedings of a Workshop was prepared by the workshop rapporteur as a factual summary of what occurred at the workshop. Statements, recommendations, and opinions expressed are those of individual presenters and participants, and are not necessarily endorsed or verified by the National Academies of Sciences, Engineering, and Medicine, and they should not be construed as reflecting any group consensus.

human capital and equal opportunity. This vision rests on the recognition that improved health outcomes are shaped by interdependent social, economic, environmental, genetic, behavioral, and health care factors and will require robust national and community-based policies and dependable resources to achieve that vision. The roundtable recognizes that rural health is part of the population health narrative and aims to explore and better understand rural health issues.

WORKSHOP OBJECTIVES

The workshop was structured to follow the institutionally approved Statement of Task (see Box 1-1). Divided into five sessions held over 2 days, the workshop featured invited presentations and discussion that focused on:

- rural America in context,
- rural health vital signs,
- rural health care in action,
- assessment and implementation strategies for improving the health of rural populations, and
- rural health policy.

The workshop began with setting the context and assessing current measures of rural health, and then the scope was expanded to discuss rural health care assessment, strategy, and implementation along with rural health policy. In accordance with the policies of the National Academies, the workshop did not attempt to establish any conclusions or develop recommendations about needs and future directions, focusing instead on issues identified by the speakers and workshop participants.

BOX 1-1
Statement of Task

A planning committee of the National Academies of Sciences, Engineering, and Medicine will organize and convene a public workshop to explore population health in rural America. The workshop will host speakers from sectors that contribute to population health in rural communities, such as health care, public health, and community-based organizations. Presentations will highlight promising activities attributable to each sector that contribute to improving population health. A proceedings of the presentations and discussion at the workshop will be prepared by a designated rapporteur in accordance with institutional guidelines.

The proceedings of the presentations and discussions held at the workshop was prepared by a designated rapporteur in accordance with institutional guidelines.

ORGANIZATION OF THE PROCEEDINGS

The proceedings of this workshop is organized into six chapters. Chapter 2, Rural America in Context, provides an overview of rural demographics and a framework for discussing the infrastructure challenges in rural areas. Chapter 3, Rural Health Vital Signs, offers insights into public health in rural settings, including key measures of mortality and morbidity in rural areas, tribal public health activities, and rural health indicators. Chapter 4, Rural Health Care in Action, explores the landscape of rural health, the state of tribal health care in rural settings, the implications of wraparound services for rural America, and the role of community health workers in rural health. Chapter 5, Assessment and Implementation Strategies for Improving the Health of Rural Populations, examines assessment and implementation strategies for rural population health. Chapter 6, Rural Health Policy, presents the current state of rural health policy and explores the opportunities for improving rural health through policy. The speaker and planning committee members biosketches are in Appendix A, the workshop agenda is in Appendix B, and the references are in Appendix C.

2

Rural America in Context

The first session of the workshop focused on providing context, including the demographics and social determinants of health (SDOH) in rural America, as well as the effect of structural urbanism on health care access and delivery and other challenges related to the health care infrastructure in rural areas. The session was moderated by Lars Peterson from the Rural & Underserved Health Research Center at the University of Kentucky.

RURAL DEMOGRAPHICS AND SOCIAL DETERMINANTS OF HEALTH

Alana Knudson from the Walsh Center for Rural Health Analysis at NORC at the University of Chicago highlighted relevant demographic features of rural communities in the United States. SDOH—including poverty, unemployment, lack of affordable housing, and food insecurity—are challenges facing rural America. She noted that SDOH intersect with race and age, putting some rural subgroups at greater risk for unmet needs, including children, African Americans, and Native Americans.

Demographics of Rural America

Knudson provided an overview of the demographics of rural America, which differ substantially from urban America in terms of age distribution, race, ethnicity, and the effects of migration. Approximately 60 million people in the United States—representing about one-fifth of the national population—live in rural areas.[1]

Older Adults in Rural and Nonrural Areas

A striking difference between rural and urban populations is reflected in their age distributions, said Knudson. Forty years ago, the percentage of Americans aged 65 years and older was smaller in rural areas than in urban settings. However, the past four decades have seen a dramatic shift in those proportions, with older adults now representing approximately 18 percent of the rural population and 14 percent of the urban population.[2] As of 2016, almost one out of every five rural residents was aged 65 years or older. This demographic shift toward older populations creates both opportunities and challenges for rural communities. In this respect, it is relevant to consider the areas where older adults in rural areas tend to reside in the United States. Knudson added that in 2017, most rural counties in which more than 20 percent of the population was aged 65 years or older were located in scenic areas or areas with chronic population loss (see Figure 2-1).[3] Many older Americans retire in rural areas that are recreation or retirement destinations. Additionally, many rural counties have had persistent population loss over the past 40 years attributable to younger people migrating from rural communities to urban areas in search of jobs. In geographical terms, the distribution of rural elderly populations is somewhat different than in metropolitan (metro)[4] communities. This is evident in the concentration of counties with a high proportion of older residents in the central Great Plains and in the West, she added.

---

[1] More information about rural America is available at https://gis-portal.data.census.gov/arcgis/apps/MapSeries/index.html?appid=7a41374f6b03456e9d138cb014711e01 (accessed August 6, 2020).

[2] Rural population data from U.S. Census. More information about U.S. Census data is available at https://data.census.gov/cedsci (accessed July 17, 2020).

[3] Rural county data from the Economic Research Service at the U.S. Department of Agriculture. For more information about rural county data, see https://www.ers.usda.gov (accessed July 17, 2020).

[4] Knudson noted that a challenge in rural health research is that *rural* is often referred to as *nonmetro*, as is the case with the data from the U.S. Department of Agriculture. She added that some rural health researchers would like to shift that terminology by comparing *rural* and *nonrural* areas.

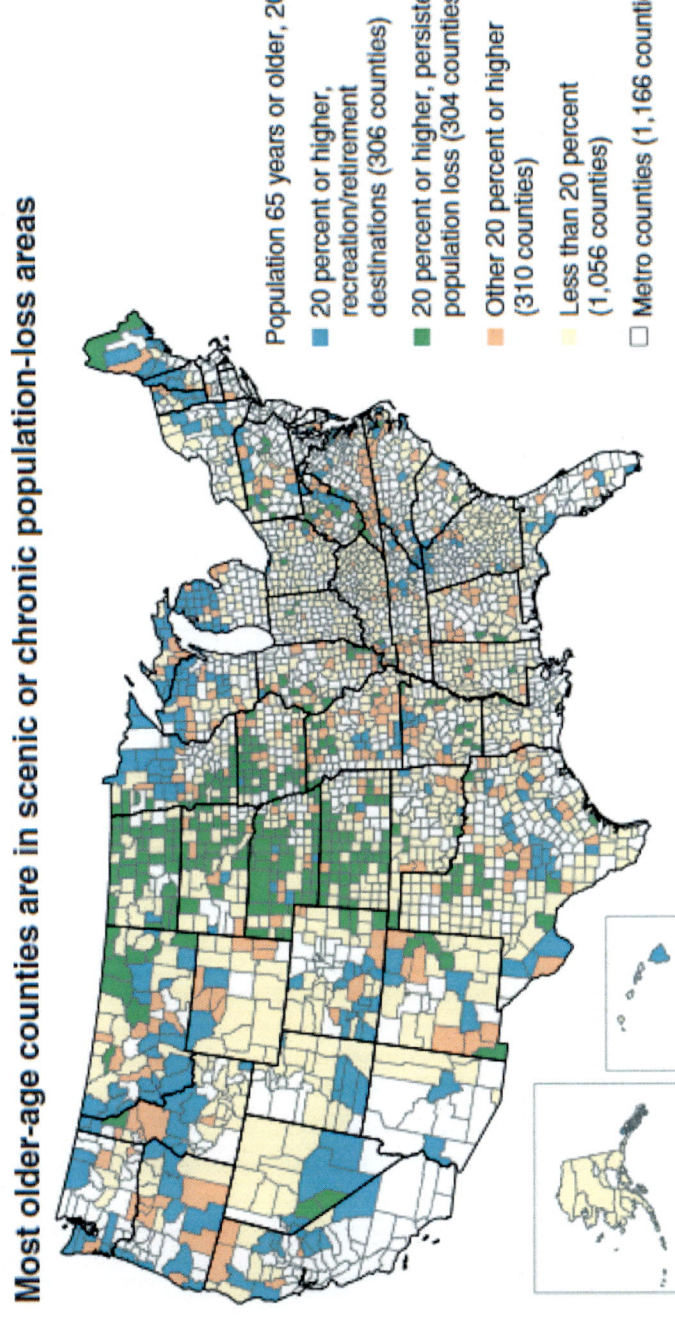

FIGURE 2-1 Rural counties with more than 20 percent of their populations aged 65 years or older, 2017.
SOURCES: Knudson presentation, June 24, 2020; Economic Research Service at the U.S. Department of Agriculture using data from the U.S. Census Bureau Population Estimates program.

Race and Ethnicity in Rural and Nonrural Areas

Stark differences between rural and nonrural populations also emerge when looking at race and ethnicity, said Knudson. For instance, metro areas tend to have higher concentrations of racial and ethnic minorities. According to 2017 data, nonwhite residents made up about 42 percent of the metro population compared to 22 percent of the rural population (Cromartie, 2018). Racial and ethnic differences in rural populations also emerge when analyzed by age distribution, she added.

Knudson described sociodemographic information from 2012 to 2015 on the sociodemographic characteristics of adults aged 18 years or more in rural areas in the United States by race and ethnicity. She explained that more non-Hispanic whites (25.7 percent) aged 65 and older were living in rural areas than other racial and ethnic groups (non-Hispanic Blacks: 17.4 percent; American Indians and Alaska Natives: 13.7 percent; Hispanics: 8.6 percent; Asians and Native Hawaiians or other Pacific Islanders: 7.5 percent) (James et al., 2017). In contrast, more Hispanic adults (66.0 percent) aged 18–44 were living in rural areas than other racial and ethnic groups (Asians and Native Hawaiians or other Pacific Islanders: 60.5 percent; Native Americans/Alaska Natives: 49.3 percent; non-Hispanic Blacks: 43.7 percent; non-Hispanic whites: 36.9 percent) (see Figure 2-2). Knudson noted that over the past 20 years, the greatest growth in racial and ethnic representation in rural communities has occurred among the Hispanic, American Indian, and Alaska Native populations.

Effect of Migration

Knudson explained that changes in migration patterns have also occurred across the country in the past decade.[5] Many of the rural areas that have seen an increase in net migration rates are destination areas with recreational opportunities, particularly in the West, which are areas that also tend to draw people moving or relocating for retirement. Changes in employment opportunities have also led to migration shifts. For example, population changes from 2012 to 2013 and from 2016 to 2017 correspond to shifts in energy extraction in areas such as the northern part of North Dakota and the eastern Montana border, where a change in oil prices led to the evaporation of jobs and subsequently to a large loss of population. Knudson noted that another shift is ongoing in response to the coronavirus disease 2019 (COVID-19) pandemic, with some urban residents leaving for second homes located in rural areas. She noted that as people

---

[5] Rural net migration patterns from the Economic Research Service at the U.S. Department of Agriculture using data from the U.S. Census Bureau Population Estimates program. More information is available at https://www.ers.usda.gov (accessed July 17, 2020).

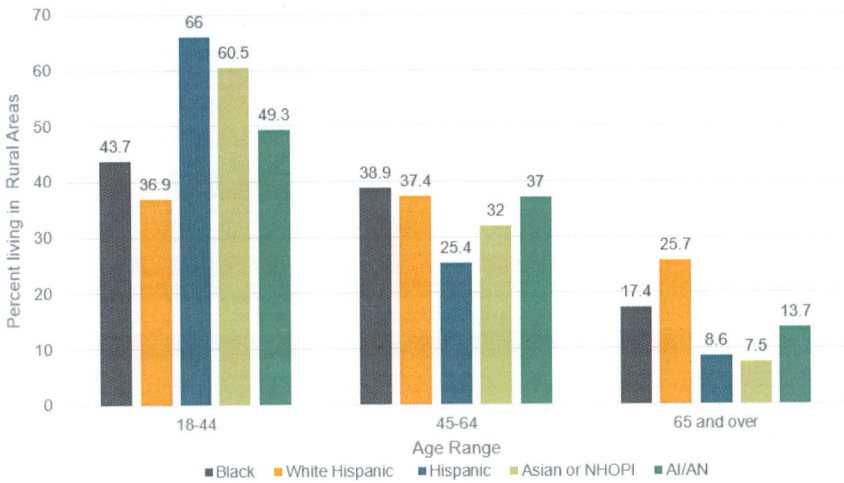

FIGURE 2-2 Race and ethnicity in rural areas.
NOTE: AI/AN = American Indian/Alaska Native; NHOPI = Native Hawaiian or other Pacific Islander.
SOURCE: Knudson Presentation, June 23, 2020.

demonstrate that it is possible to successfully work remotely, many may decide to reside primarily outside of the larger urban areas. Knudson suggested that in 4 years, the migration map may look different because of COVID-19.

Social Determinants of Health

Knudson explained that in the domain of public health, the SDOH are often conceptualized in terms of where people live, learn, work, play, and pray and how those factors contribute to people's health and well-being. Specifically, the SDOH are the neighborhood and built environment, health and health care, the social and community context, education, and economic stability.[6] To explore the effect of economic stability on the health and well-being of people in rural areas, she noted that "wealth equals health." Earning a livable wage with compensation that enables access to affordable health care and health insurance is a foundational component of good health and well-being.

---

[6] Categories of SDOH as defined by the Office of Disease Prevention and Health Promotion are available at https://www.healthypeople.gov/2020/topics-objectives/topic/social-determinants-of-health (accessed July 21, 2020).

Trends in employment rates from 2007 to 2019 differ in rural and urban areas, said Knudson.[7] During the economic recession from late 2007 to mid-2009, rural and urban employment rates were comparable. By 2014, urban employment rates had rebounded to prerecession levels. However, growth in rural employment rates has been slower to rebound; by 2019, the rates had not yet reached the 2007 levels. The COVID-19 pandemic is continuing to harm small businesses, which will likely pose additional challenges to achieving prerecession employment levels in rural areas. Similarly, rural areas have struggled to achieve reductions in poverty rates that have been attained in metro areas, said Knudson. The mid-20th century saw a sizeable decrease in the nonmetro poverty rate, which dropped from 33.2 percent to 17.9 percent between 1959 and 1969.[8] However, rural communities have never attained the same level of affluence as urban communities.

In 2018, the poverty rate for nonmetro residents was 16.1 percent compared to 12.6 percent for metro residents. Poverty rates vary in different rural areas across the country, with greater percentages of rural communities living in poverty concentrated in Appalachia, along the Mississippi Delta, in some areas of border states, in areas in the West predominantly populated by American Indian tribal communities, and in Alaska Native communities.[9] Rural communities are also disproportionately affected by persistent poverty, which has long-lasting implications for health and well-being, she added. Counties with persistent poverty are those in which at least 20 percent of county residents have been poor for the previous four decades.[10] Concentrations of rural counties experiencing persistent poverty are found in Appalachia, in the South, along the Mississippi Delta, along the U.S.–Mexico border, and tribal lands inhabited by American Indians and Alaska Natives.

Knudson described how racial and ethnic disparities intersect with geographic disparities in wealth. In 2018, rural residents who were African American, American Indian, or Alaska Native experienced the highest

---

[7] Rural and urban employment data from the Economic Research Service at the U.S. Department of Agriculture using data from the Local Area Unemployment Statistics at the U.S. Bureau of Labor Statistics. More information is available at https://www.ers.usda.gov (accessed July 17, 2020).

[8] More information on poverty and well-being is available at https://www.ers.usda.gov/topics/rural-economy-population/rural-poverty-well-being/#historic (accessed July 17, 2020).

[9] See https://www.census.gov/data-tools/demo/saipe/#/?map_geoSelector=aa_c (accessed November 28, 2020).

[10] More information on populations in poverty by county is available at https://www.census.gov/data-tools/demo/saipe/#/?map_geoSelector=aa_c (accessed July 17, 2020).

rates of poverty among people in the United States.[11] Across all racial and ethnic populations, a greater percentage of rural residents live in poverty compared to their urban counterparts. This trend also presents in poverty rates among children under the age of 5 years, with 25 percent of those children living in poverty in rural areas compared to 18.6 percent in urban areas.[12] Across the entire continuum of age distributions, greater percentages of rural residents live in poverty than urban residents. Residents of rural communities also tend to face challenges with respect to food security and housing affordability, she noted. People living more than 30 miles from a grocery store are considered to have low access to grocery stores.[13] The highest percentages of people with low grocery store access are concentrated in central and western parts of the country, which are areas that tend to be more sparsely populated. Similarly, central and western rural regions feature some of the least affordable housing options based on the ratio of housing prices to income.[14] The Walsh Center for Rural Health Analysis at NORC at the University of Chicago looked at the ability of Missouri residents to maintain housing and found that although housing prices were affordable, the cost of electricity was not. This is one example of the multiple factors that determine whether rural residents are able to maintain safe and affordable housing.

Knudson remarked that many challenges faced by rural America can be addressed through innovative local solutions that leverage the strong resilience of many rural communities. Among ongoing efforts is the Rural Health Information Hub, which provides comprehensive tool kits to address the SDOH in rural communities.[15]

---

[11] Poverty rates by metro and nonmetro residence from the Economic Research Service at the U.S. Department of Agriculture. More information on poverty and well-being is available at https://www.ers.usda.gov/topics/rural-economy-population/rural-poverty-well-being/#historic (accessed July 17, 2020).

[12] Poverty rates by age and metro and nonmetro residence from the Economic Research Service at the U.S. Department of Agriculture. More information on poverty and well-being is available at https://www.ers.usda.gov/topics/rural-economy-population/rural-poverty-well-being/#historic (accessed July 17, 2020).

[13] Data on grocery store access from the Economic Research Service at the U.S. Department of Agriculture. More information is available at https://www.ers.usda.gov/data-products/food-environment-atlas/go-to-the-atlas (accessed July 17, 2020).

[14] More information on rural housing affordability is available at https://oregoneconomicanalysis.com/2017/02/09/rural-housing-affordability (accessed July 17, 2020).

[15] Additional information from the Rural Health Information Hub and the Social Determinants of Health in Rural Communities Toolkit can be found at https://www.ruralhealthinfo.org/toolkits/sdoh (accessed November 28, 2020).

STRUCTURAL URBANISM IN RURAL AMERICA

Janice Probst from the Rural & Minority Health Research Center at the Arnold School of Public Health at the University of South Carolina discussed mortality rates and race-based health disparities in rural America. She stated that data on rural communities should be examined with an awareness of "structural urbanism," a framework for addressing health issues that unintentionally and systematically discriminates against rural populations. Probst explained how structural urbanism and current funding mechanisms systematically disadvantage rural populations and negatively affect their health outcomes.

Effect of Structural Urbanism on Direct Health Care Services

Probst said that structural urbanism underlies the health issues facing rural areas. She defined this concept as "a bias toward large population centers that emerges from a focus on individuals rather than infrastructure when designing health care and public health interventions." For example, proposals for programs currently receiving public attention, such as Medicaid expansion and Medicare for All, tend to focus on individual needs rather than on infrastructure and population-level needs. One of the last major investments in health services infrastructure was the Hill-Burton program, which was in effect from 1946 to 1997 and funded the construction of hospitals and other health care facilities based on community need. The focus since then has almost exclusively centered on extending the ability of individuals to pay for care, she noted. The Medicare and Medicaid programs of 1965, the Patient Protection and Affordable Care Act of 2010, and the 2014 Medicaid expansion were all designed to provide *individuals* with the ability to acquire health care. Whether the programs were aimed at covering fee-for-service or capitation, each focused on providing the ability to acquire health care one individual at a time, rather than building health care infrastructure.

Probst asserted that funding mechanisms reimbursing direct health care services provided to individuals will never serve small populations fairly—this includes funding mechanisms relating to Medicare for All, capitation, value-based care, and other health system "tweaks" that may be proposed to address rural health. For instance, the Medicare Payment Advisory Commission has deemed home health care providers to be an inefficient service delivery model due to the long drive times between patients (MedPAC, 2017). The characteristics of rural populations make adequate service delivery within the current system's structure unattainable, Probst added.

The focus on providing health care to individuals fails because of problems of scale and undermines the provision of health care and public health services in rural settings, said Probst. Most health care models, including fee-for-service and capitation models, require a minimum number of funded participants to be viable under current financing mechanisms. Sparsely populated rural areas are at a disadvantage in systems that operate on scale. Similarly, public health's focus on national goals obscures local problems and small populations. Because of the requirements for a minimum number of funded participants and the focus on attaining national goals, rural communities are often excluded from public health programs, she explained.

Probst noted that some resources contend that a physician's office in a private-pay health care system requires an estimated 1,900–2,500 patients to operate successfully.[16] Small populations generally cannot provide this number of patients to a single office, which discourages practitioners from opening offices in rural areas. Metropolitan counties in the United States have an average of 53 primary care physicians per 100,000 people, but rural counties average just 39 physicians per 100,000 people.[17] Probst suggested that this type of à la carte system through which individuals purchase health care one service at a time results in a lack of care for people who need it in some geographic areas. An example of this health care shortage in rural areas is the limited availability of intensive care units (ICUs) in many areas. In response to rising concerns about the lack of ICU beds amid the COVID-19 pandemic, the Kaiser Family Foundation (KFF) and Kaiser Health news mapped the availability of ICU beds by county across the rural regions of America. The geographic analysis revealed that numerous counties either have only hospitals without ICU beds or no hospitals at all.[18] It has been argued that small counties may not require their own hospitals or hospitals with ICU beds, she noted. However, the effect of structural urbanism also extends to smaller, billable services such as education activities for patients with chronic conditions.

---

[16] The presenter provided the following resource as a reference: https://www.medicaleconomics.com/view/6-keys-profitability (accessed October 28, 2020).

[17] More information about rural health care workforce shortages, socioeconomic factors, and health inequity is available at https://www.ruralhealthweb.org/about-nrha/about-rural-health-care (accessed July 31, 2020).

[18] More information is available at https://khn.org/news/as-coronavirus-spreads-widely-millions-of-older-americans-live-in-counties-with-no-icu-beds (accessed July 17, 2020).

Effect of Structural Urbanism on Diabetes Management—an Example

The effect of lack of access to hospital care extends to the management of chronic conditions, explained Probst. Diabetes is an example of a disease that is primarily managed by patients, but treatment for diabetes is not intuitive or as simple as taking a pill—it requires the monitoring of glucose and insulin levels. Patients require education to effectively manage this disease, which is a billable service under Medicare and Medicaid, but there is a shortage of patient education programs in rural areas because the health system is funded via individualized payments. Diabetes is highly prevalent among adults in the United States, affecting approximately 9 percent of urban and 9.9 percent of rural adults. Multiple compositional factors influence health outcomes for the rural population; this results in a higher risk of death for people with diabetes who live in rural areas. These causative factors include lower levels of education and lower health insurance rates in rural America. Contextual factors emerge because the infrastructure for patient education must be built "one paying person at a time," she added. For instance, 62 percent of rural counties do not have a single diabetes management education program, even though certifying diabetes educators is fairly simple, and physicians could also be trained to provide these services (Rutledge et al., 2017).

This shortage persists despite the large burden of diabetes in many regions across the United States, with death rates higher for rural residents with diabetes across racial and ethnic groups. According to 2017–2018 data, for example, adults with diabetes living in rural areas had an age-adjusted death rate per 100,000 population that was 46 percent higher than their urban counterparts for people aged 25–64 years and about 24 percent higher for adults aged 65 years or older, according to Probst's analysis of Centers for Disease Control and Prevention (CDC) data.[19] These disparities in death rates for people in urban versus rural areas also extend to racial and ethnic minorities. Probst contended that although the lack of diabetes education programs is not the sole cause for this increased risk of mortality, greater local availability of certified diabetes educators—which could be achieved by simply training existing physicians—could help address this issue.

---

[19] Author's analysis of data from CDC Wide-ranging Online Data for Epidemiologic Research (WONDER): Centers for Disease Control and Prevention, National Center for Health Statistics. Underlying Cause of Death 2017–2018 on CDC WONDER Online Database, released in 2020. Data are from the Multiple Cause of Death Files, as compiled from data provided by the 57 vital statistics jurisdictions through the Vital Statistics Cooperative Program. See http://wonder.cdc.gov/ucd-icd10.html (accessed June 9, 2020).

Effect of Structural Urbanism on Public Health

Rural Visibility in National Data

The shortcomings of approaches that focus on individuals apply to public health as well, said Probst. Health outcomes in rural areas often have poor visibility in national-level data. For instance, national goals set by large agencies, such as the Healthy People 2020 agenda, often feature national averages without the analysis of subgroup data that is needed to accurately assess the success of public health initiatives. To illustrate, Probst noted that the Healthy People 2020 national targets for child mortality had been met for four out of five age groups by 2017 (Khan et al., 2018). Without examining subgroup data, it appears that efforts to reduce child mortality rates have been successful. However, analysis of mortality rates for rural youth—which are higher than national averages—reveals that the Healthy People 2020 targets had not been achieved for youth in any of the five age brackets (Probst et al., 2019).

Plans for national success based on aggregate individual-level data neglect rural surveillance, said Probst. For example, CDC's *Health, United States, 2017* report contains 144 tables, but only 19 percent presented outcomes for rural populations (NCHS, 2018). In addition to the lack of rural surveillance, a focus on numbers instead of severity restricts rural opportunities for improvement. For instance, during the 2015 HIV outbreak in Scott County, Indiana, 150 people contracted HIV/AIDS. This translates to a population-based statistic of 630 per 100,000 people, which was well above the national average of 421 per 100,000 in 2016 (Gonsalves and Crawford, 2018). Looking only at case numbers masks the high rate of infection in such a small county. Funding restrictions further limit opportunities to improve rural health, said Probst. South Carolina faced challenges in competing for the 2011–2014 CDC community transformation grants because eligibility required a minimum population of 500,000. This grant structure excluded rural areas and required the development of a program proposal to serve the entire state in order to be eligible to bid.

Effect of COVID-19 on Structural Challenges in Rural Care

The COVID-19 pandemic has intensified these structural problems, said Probst. Small health care facilities in rural areas are facing substantial economic hardships because of declining person-based payments. Community health centers have reported declines of income of 70–80 percent (Wright et al., 2021). Stay-at-home orders associated with the COVID-19 pandemic have resulted in a nationwide decline in physician office visits (Rubin, 2020), and some rural hospitals have needed to furlough staff because of the decline in elective procedures.[20] She noted that smaller facilities have been disproportionately affected by declining person-based payments and declining physician office visits, and the person-based payment system in the United States provides no clear path to recovery for rural health facilities. When rural hospitals and physician offices close, there are no mechanisms to bring these jobs and services back to the communities they serve after the pandemic. Probst warned that without substantial changes to the ways that rural health care is delivered and funded, the COVID-19 pandemic could potentially decimate rural America's entire health infrastructure.

Health Care as Infrastructure: Framework for Change

As a framework for change to address the barriers posed by structural urbanism, Probst suggested framing health care as essential infrastructure within a community. To illustrate, she contrasted the support provided to small, underresourced communities to develop transportation and power infrastructures with the lack of support those communities receive to develop health infrastructure. Loving County, Texas, has 169 residents and could not afford to pave its own roads or build electrical infrastructure without state and national funding support, which is provided because state and local governments recognize that these services are essential for all communities regardless of whether counties can afford them independently. Probst maintained that health care should be similarly framed as essential community infrastructure required for residents' health and well-being, rather than as a discretionary purchase made by an individual. This paradigm shift would construe health care as (1) a characteristic of a community rather than a service accessed by an individual, (2) responsive to community needs, and (3) funded as a utility via taxation and/or regulated fees that maintain services for all populations in need. Changing the funding mechanisms would shift determinations about service provision. Under a framework where health was funded as a utility, a hospital that would previously have been considered "not viable under current, centrally determined rates" would not be closed. Instead, reimbursement rates would be sufficient to maintain the institution's viability, and communities would continue to have access to the health care services it provides. This new framework would also help to protect industry in smaller communities, added Probst. Many companies are reluctant to operate in areas without hospitals because the lack of

---

[20] More information about rural hospital staff furlough is available at https://www.beckershospitalreview.com/finance/10-hospitals-furloughing-staff-in-response-to-covid-19.html (accessed July 17, 2020).

hospital access complicates emergency care access and thus may affect worker's compensation requirements.

Probst acknowledged the difficulties involved in such a fundamental shift in the framework for health care delivery and funding. For instance, determining how to allocate funding and determine the levels of need can be challenging and contentious, even in countries with central health services, such as Great Britain. Additionally, defining the geographic coverage areas for supporting health care is complex—it can be done by state, region, or a combination. For instance, the Tennessee Valley Authority covers parts of seven states, while the Delta Valley Authority includes eight states within the Mississippi Delta.[21] Despite the challenges involved in driving change, "the consequences of failure to strengthen the faltering rural health care infrastructure would be much worse," said Probst. She then added that the United States will not be internationally competitive without a strong rural base for extractive and small manufacturing industries. Rural health care is in decline, and the communities that lose their health infrastructure are often the communities that are most in need. A focus on communities and building their health infrastructure offers one path forward, she said.

DISCUSSION

Funding Health Care as a Utility

The discussion section of the session was moderated by Lars Peterson, who shared impressions and posed questions from the public. Peterson remarked that one of the issues facing rural hospitals is a higher fixed cost for low patient volumes, which can lead to hospital closures. He asked Probst if the model she outlined would provide subsidies or enhanced payments to low-volume hospitals. While other mechanisms may be feasible, Probst said that the mechanism she envisions is that of enhanced payments, but these payments must be thought of in a new manner. She drew a comparison between health care and public education. Every state constitution requires education to be provided to all children, with a mixture of local and state funds allocated to schools. Without this mixed-funding stream, rural schools would not be viable. Rural hospitals encounter higher fixed costs because of the need for hospitals to be a certain size and the relatively smaller patient populations in rural areas. In education, similar challenges have been addressed by

---

[21] See Tennessee Valley Authority, *About TVA*, available at https://www.tva.com/about-tva (accessed October 28, 2020), and Delta Regional Authority, *DRA States*, available at https://dra.gov/about-dra/dra-states (accessed October 28, 2020).

treating education as a utility. Probst emphasized that building electrical infrastructure in small counties is not cost-effective, but the need for such infrastructure is broadly accepted. Thus, she advocates for a new funding mechanism that would treat health care as a public utility.

She said that the current health infrastructure model provides no control over hospital location; hospitals are free to close or relocate at will. In contrast, electric companies are regulated utilities that cannot opt to cease serving rural areas. Peterson brought up the issue of state funding of roads, with states sometimes allocating funds to larger population centers instead of rural areas. He asked whether restructuring health care as infrastructure might lead to urban areas receiving better maintained facilities than rural areas. Probst acknowledged that to be a risk but noted that at least there is a political process for such issues to be addressed, unlike a system managed by private equity companies in which citizens have no voice.

Challenges and Opportunities of Age-Based Migration

Citing Knudson's demographic data regarding the higher concentration of older adults in rural areas resulting from youth migration, Peterson asked her to expound on the associated opportunities and challenges. Knudson replied that the lack of an adequate health care workforce to support the population's needs is a challenge faced by communities with a higher proportion of older adults. To illustrate, she described a rural hospital in North Dakota that closed its nursing home wing, in spite of having a waiting list of potential residents, because of a workforce shortage of certified nursing assistants and licensed practical nurses. However, she pointed out that communities with larger proportions of older adults also present valuable opportunities. The types of intergenerational settings emerging in some retirement destinations have communities in which people are integrated across the age spectrum. For example, some health care training programs are collocated with residential facilities for older adults, which provides opportunities for multigenerational learning and exchange. Knudson suggested shifting from a deficit-focused view of older Americans to an asset-focused view that acknowledges the contributions older populations make to the fabric of their communities.

Telehealth Services

Peterson asked about the potential interplay between the lack of diabetes patient education programs described by Probst and the increase in telecommuting work that Knudson mentioned. He queried whether the lack of broadband availability in rural areas could limit the implementation of telehealth in those areas and perhaps feed into structural urbanism and worsen disparities. Probst replied that telehealth could be helpful for medical services that do not require a physical exam, such as follow-up appointments and psychiatric consultations, but she acknowledged that sufficient broadband capacity is still not in place. Knudson suggested that one way to categorize rural communities is by the availability of broadband services. She expects broadband to play a greater role in health care moving forward, so the assessment of broadband access could help define who has access to health care and who does not.

Rural Terminology and County Size

A virtual participant asked for clarification of the terms *metro*, *nonmetro*, *rural*, and *urban* and noted that data are often presented at the county level, but county size varies hugely across the nation. Knudson explained that there are many definitions of the term *rural*, with some currently used definitions going back to the 1800s when the landscape of infrastructure was very different (Mueller et al., 2020). She also noted that the broad variation in county sizes across the country—some counties in the western United States are as large as the states of Connecticut, Massachusetts, and Rhode Island combined—can limit apt comparisons of county-level data and assessment of infrastructure needs. Generally, counties with less than 50,000 people are categorized as rural, and counties with more than 50,000 people are categorized as urban, although some policy makers have pushed to raise the threshold for the urban designation to 500,000. Knudson suggested that population per square mile would be a better metric for assessing access to health care. Probst expressed similar concern about defining counties with less than 500,000 people as rural, because solving the problems of structural urbanism will require assessing the needs of rural communities with finer granularity. She noted that mechanisms such as the Health Professional Shortage Areas do consider multiple factors such as population, population health, and the availability of health providers,[22] but even those definitions can be contentious.

Factors Affecting Access to Rural Health Care

Peterson asked whether there is a cultural or behavioral element to health care access in rural areas, noting the perception (accurate or not) that rural populations are more self-reliant and prefer to address health

---

[22] For more information, see https://bhw.hrsa.gov/shortage-designation/hpsas (accessed August 13, 2020).

concerns on their own when possible. He asked whether such a culture might explain delayed care that leads to the development of more severe conditions. Peterson asked whether a relationship between a culture of self-reliance and a delay in accessing care has been observed anecdotally or in research, as well as whether rural culture may contribute to health disparities.

Probst explained that there is not a singular rural culture—there are multiple rural cultures across the country. Tangible factors such as "travel impedance" play a role in how promptly people can access care. Citing her own experiences growing up in a rural area, Probst drew a comparison to shopping. Her family did not go to the store frequently because of travel impedance, waiting until there was a real need for items rather than a mere desire. Similarly, as a health condition becomes more severe, the need to seek care tends to outweigh the burden of travel impedance. Cost of care is also a factor, said Probst. She contended that what some people may view as cultural individualism may actually be a response to the high cost of health care for individuals who have high deductible health insurance policies or no insurance at all. Knudson added that rural residents have historically had lower rates of health insurance coverage. She surmised that perhaps because of how closely knit some communities are, people may prefer not to owe money to anyone in their community, so the decision to forgo health care may be as much a financial preference as it is a cultural preference.

3

Rural Health Vital Signs

The second session of the workshop featured presentations on the drivers of the rural–urban gap in mortality rates, the health effects related to the extent of racial and ethnic disparities within rural communities, and public health challenges faced by Alaska Native tribal communities. Presenters also provided an overview of the Department of Health and Human Services' (HHS's) ongoing Healthy People and Rural Healthy People initiatives. The session was moderated by Alana Knudson from the Walsh Center for Rural Health Analysis at NORC at the University of Chicago.

WHY IS MORTALITY HIGHER IN RURAL AMERICA?

Mark Holmes from the North Carolina Rural Health Research and Policy Analysis Center at the University of North Carolina at Chapel Hill discussed the rural–urban gap in mortality rates and explored the drivers of these geographic disparities. He also discussed the policy implications of these drivers and the initial trends of the coronavirus disease 2019 (COVID-19) pandemic in terms of rurality, morbidity, and mortality.

Rural–Urban Mortality Gap

Holmes described the rural–urban mortality gap, which is characterized by higher mortality rates in rural (nonmetro) areas than in urban (metro) areas.[1] Although this rural–urban mortality gap varies across regions, it has been increasing overall and is attributable to drivers that include access to health services, population behaviors, and the social determinants of health (SDOH). The gap in age-adjusted mortality between metro and nonmetro areas in the United States has widened over the past decade, even as overall mortality has been decreasing (see Figure 3-1). Between 1999 and 2008, the gap held steady at about 7 percent, with mortality in both metro and nonmetro populations decreasing at roughly the same rate. However, these two trends began to diverge in 2009, when mortality rates continued to decline steadily in metro areas but the rates began to increase in nonmetro areas. By 2016, the gap between metro and nonmetro areas had almost tripled to 19 percent.

Drivers of Higher Mortality in Nonmetro Areas

Holmes described how specific drivers of higher mortality may account for divergent mortality trends in metro versus nonmetro areas. An analysis of the trends in metro and nonmetro mortality data from 1980 to 2010 found that county demographics, economics, and geographic distribution in each decade explained the growing rural–urban health gap (Spencer et al., 2018). In 1980, mortality rates in metro and nonmetro areas were approximately the same. The rural–urban mortality gap began to emerge between 1980 and 1990, and the gap continued to expand between 2000 and 2010. By hypothetically adjusting rural counties to have the same population demographics as urban counties—but retaining much of the existing rural infrastructure—the researchers found that the age-adjusted mortality rate in the rural counties with urban demographics dropped to the same rate as urban counties. This demonstrates that demographics and economics are increasing predictors of the rural–urban mortality gap, he said (Spencer et al., 2018).

Behavior is another driver of the rural–urban mortality gap, said Holmes. Modifiable risk factors such as smoking, obesity, and excessive alcohol use lead to higher rates of death attributable to certain potentially preventable conditions (e.g., acute myocardial infarction, lung cancer, diabetes, stroke, chronic obstructive pulmonary disease [COPD]). Holmes noted that both smoking and obesity rates tend to be higher in rural areas (19.1 and 31.5 percent, respectively) than in urban areas (15.8 and 26.7 percent, respectively), while rates of excessive alcohol use are higher in urban areas (Holmes and Thompson, 2019). This

---

[1] Holmes explained that the designations of metro areas as urban and of nonmetro areas as rural is based on county population thresholds. Counties that are close to the upper bound of the population threshold are generally considered to be metro areas.

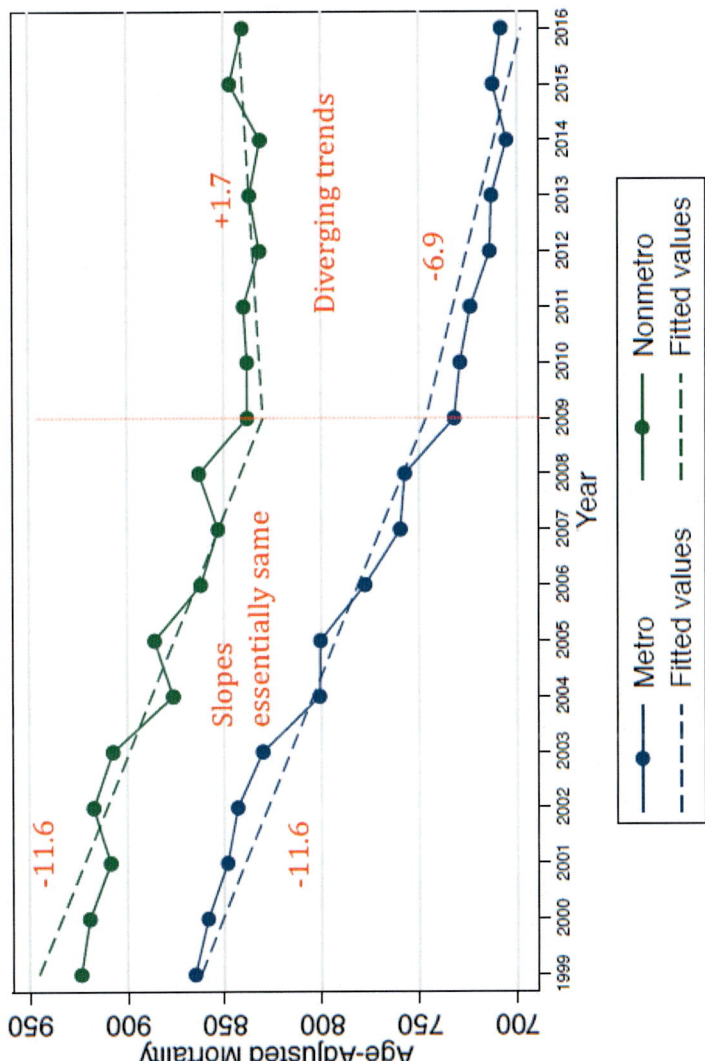

FIGURE 3-1 Diverging trends in age-adjusted mortality in metro versus nonmetro areas in the United States.
SOURCES: Holmes presentation, June 24, 2020; data from Centers for Disease Control and Prevention WONDER (Wide-ranging Online Data for Epidemiologic Research) compressed mortality data (2013 Metro Status); see https://wonder.cdc.gov (accessed August 3, 2020).

disparity in modifiable risk factor rates suggests that rural areas have a greater percentage of potentially preventable deaths attributable to specific conditions than urban areas. Addressing those modifiable risk factors could potentially prevent more of those types of deaths in rural areas than in urban areas.

The lack of health care providers is another driver of higher mortality in rural areas, added Holmes. Rural areas tend to have fewer health care professionals per capita than urban areas. Specifically, a substantial disparity in the numbers of mental health care professionals exists between rural and urban areas (Larson et al., 2019; NCHWA, 2010; van Dis, 2002). Rural hospital closures are another contributing factor. Between 2010 and 2014, 171 rural hospitals closed in the United States; these closures were concentrated in the American South, a region widely affected by rural health issues.[2]

Variation in Causes of Death

Holmes explained that the increasing rural–urban mortality gap is being driven by certain conditions, including heart disease, unintentional injury, suicide, cirrhosis, COPD, lung cancer, and stroke (Singh and Siahpush, 2014). In his research, Holmes used U.S. Census regions and divisions to explore which causes of death are relatively more common in rural areas within each geographic region.[3] For instance, comparing the mortality from diabetes in rural New England to that of urban New England can reveal the geographically standardized rural–urban mortality gap. This type of analysis demonstrates that certain causes of death are consistently overrepresented in rural areas across the United States, including motor vehicle accidents, suicide by gun (which is relatively more common in the Northeast region), other nontransport accidents (e.g., asphyxiation), and acute myocardial infarction. Holmes explained that these trends are related to factors such as the effect of mental health on suicide by firearm and the effect of lack of timely access to trauma care on accidents and acute myocardial infarction. Thus, the overrepresentation of these causes of death in rural areas can be linked to structural drivers of mortality, such as gaps in the supply of mental health professionals and increasing closures of rural hospitals.

---

[2] More information about these rural hospital closures is available at https://www.shepscenter.unc.edu/programs-projects/rural-health/rural-hospital-closures (accessed July 6, 2020).

[3] The U.S. Census designates four geographic regions (West, Midwest, Northeast, and South) and nine regional divisions (Pacific, Mountain, West North Central, West South Central, East North Central, East South Central, New England, Middle Atlantic, and South Atlantic).

Regional variations in rural health suggest that a nationwide one-size-fits-all approach may not be the best approach to rural health policy, said Holmes. He recommended that policy makers consider which policies may improve rural health in regions with higher disparities. Additionally, policies should be shaped by an understanding of the underlying causes of variations, such as the quality of trauma health systems or the safety of highways. For instance, the Department of Transportation may be best suited to take action to address regional disparities in motor vehicle accidents.

COVID-19 Mortality in Rural Areas

Holmes noted that as of June 2020, COVID-19 mortality was lower in rural areas, with the exception of the American South. He presented data from *The New York Times* Github that compared COVID-19 cases per 100,000 across the U.S. North, Midwest, South, and West and in areas designated as metropolitan (i.e., population greater than 49,000), micropolitan (i.e., population between 10,000 and 49,000), or neither.[4] Both data sets reveal similar COVID-19 trends. Metropolitan areas in the North had the highest number of cases and deaths among all areas and regions. In the West and Midwest regions, there was a gradient from highest to lowest case and death rates in areas designated as metropolitan, micropolitan, and neither, respectively. In these regions, more urbanized areas experienced higher COVID-19 rates than less urbanized areas. Particularly sharp gradients were observed in the Midwest region among metropolitan, micropolitan, and neither areas in terms of rates of both COVID-19 cases and deaths. The South is an exception to this trend, as the amount of urbanization in areas in the South was not strongly linked to rates of COVID-19 cases or deaths. Holmes added that COVID-19 trends in the South have been consistent with the expectation that cases and deaths would rise first in more urbanized areas and then spread across less urbanized and rural areas.

TRIBAL HEALTH PERSPECTIVE

Valerie Nurr'araaluk Davidson, president of Alaska Pacific University, offered a tribal health perspective framed with the tenet "nothing about us without us." She described the Alaska Tribal Health System (ATHS) and the unique public health concerns faced by rural communities in

---

[4] Data collected on June 22, 2020. More information about *The New York Times* Github is available at https://github.com/nytimes/covid-19-data (accessed July 7, 2020).

Alaska. She also discussed how the COVID-19 pandemic has affected rural communities in Alaska.

To provide context, Nurr'araaluk Davidson described the remote conditions in which many Indigenous people in Alaska live. The average village size in Alaska is between 300 and 350 people. Her mother's family, for example, is from an Alaskan village called Kwigillingok, which is located within a region that is geographically similar in size to the state of Oregon and is home to 58 federally recognized tribes. All travel in this region occurs via river or airplane, as there are no roads connecting communities. In the summer, residents travel the river by boat and in the winter, they travel by driving on the frozen river. Nurr'araaluk Davidson remarked that although conversations about Alaska Natives and American Indian people sometimes focus on differences rather than commonalities, these groups share the same desires as all Americans: they wish for their children to be happy, healthy, and well educated and for their communities to be safe. However, because of the conditions in rural Alaska, Alaska Native people may need different approaches to realize those desires than people living in less remote conditions, such as leveraging the strong partnerships that have been developed by Alaska Pacific University (see Box 3-1).

BOX 3-1
Alaska Pacific University

Alaska Pacific University was established in 1959 by Peter Gordon Gould with a vision to honor Alaska's Indigenous heritage, exemplify excellence, and prepare paths. Alaska Pacific University is a member of the University of the Arctic and has a strategic affiliation with the Alaska Native Tribal Health Consortium, a statewide tribal health organization providing services to all 229 federally recognized tribes in Alaska and services formerly provided by the federal government through the Indian Health Service. This strategic affiliation allows Alaska Pacific University to focus on tribally driven and culturally responsive research, to support Indigenous researchers and scholars, and to focus on rural workforce issues. Alaska Pacific University is engaged in various supporting partnerships. It is partnered not only with 229 federally recognized tribes in Alaska, but also with more than 300 other tribes located throughout the United States. The university has strong supporting relationships with state and federal partners. State-level partners include the Alaska Department of Health & Social Services and the Department of Environmental Conservation. Its federal partners include the Indian Health Service, the Centers for Medicare & Medicaid Services, the Centers for Disease Control and Prevention (particularly the Arctic Investigations Unit), the Health Resources and Services Administration, the U.S. Department of Agriculture, and the Environmental Protection Agency.

SOURCES: Nurr'araaluk Davidson presentation, June 24, 2020; www.alaskapacific.edu (accessed April 9, 2021).

Alaska Tribal Health System

Most health care in Alaska is provided through the authorization of the Indian Health Service (IHS), which serves 2.6 million American Indian and Alaska Native people across the United States through IHS direct service, urban Indian health clinics, and tribally compacted services. Nurr'araaluk Davidson provided an overview of ATHS, which is a voluntary affiliation of tribes and tribal organizers providing health services to Alaska Native and American Indian people. The ATHS is governed by the Alaska Tribal Health Compact, which is negotiated annually with the Secretary of HHS. With approximately 12,000 employees, ATHS has a presence in every Alaskan community and essentially serves as the public health system of Alaska. Each of those tribal health organizations is autonomous and serves a specific geographic area. Together, the ATHS affiliation serves a vast geographic area that extends across the state of Alaska and is comparable in size to the entire Midwest region of the continental United States. The ATHS referral system provides a four-tier health care delivery system that includes approximately 200 rural health clinics, multiple regional hospitals, and tertiary care at the two level II trauma centers in the state of Alaska, which are located in Anchorage and Providence. She added that many tribes in Alaska and across the country are moving toward tribal self-governance—rather than governance at the state or national level—in order to address the emerging needs of communities and make agile decisions to address those needs.

Tribal Public Health Challenges

Nurr'araaluk Davidson explained that the overall health status of American Indian and Alaska Native people is far worse than that of the overall U.S. population. At the national level, the life expectancy for Alaska Native and American Indian people is 5.5 years lower than that of the general population, at 73.0 years versus 78.5 years. The leading causes of death among American Indian and Alaska Native people in the United States are heart disease, malignant neoplasm, unintentional injury, and diabetes. In Alaska, the life expectancy is even lower for American Indian and Alaska Native people, at 70.7 years, and the leading causes of death for American Indian and Alaska Native people in the state are cancer, heart disease, and unintentional injury. One area of particular public health concern in Alaska is the lack of adequate sanitation facilities, she noted. Around one-quarter of rural homes in Alaska lack running water, and honey buckets are commonly used in lieu of toilets.[5]

---

[5] Nurr'araaluk Davidson described the common use of honey buckets: "[A honey bucket] has nothing to do with honey. It is basically a toilet seat on top of a five-gallon bucket. That is how we use the restroom."

A study by the Alaska Native Tribal Health Consortium and the Centers for Disease Control and Prevention (CDC) looked at infants in Alaskan communities without access to adequate sanitation facilities (Hennessy et al., 2008). Infants in Alaskan communities without adequate sanitation facilities in the Bethel area, for example, were found to be 11 times more likely to be hospitalized for respiratory infections and 5 times more likely to be hospitalized for skin infections,[6] which typically requires them to be transported by medical evacuation (medevac) transportation to the nearest hospital facility. Nurr'araaluk Davidson emphasized that hospitalization in rural Alaska is quite different from the typical process of hospitalization throughout much of the United States. Ambulances and 911 services are unavailable in rural communities, so families must call a health clinic to initiate the hospitalization process and wait for a plane to arrive. In rural Alaska, medevac and hospitalization services may cost between $50,000 and $250,000 depending on the services that are needed. She added that each year, one-third of the infants in a rural Alaskan community will require such medevac and hospitalization services—a number she deemed unacceptable.

Nurr'araaluk Davidson remarked that the public health challenges in rural Alaska have been best addressed when care has been provided close to individuals' homes, in a culturally appropriate manner, and in languages that the rural communities understand. This has been achieved through a variety of community-based services. For instance, the Community Health Aide Program is an Alaska-specific provider type that is federally certified by IHS. Professionals in this program receive up to 2 years of training to provide a variety of services, including immunizations and prenatal exams. Without the Community Health Aide Program, Alaska would not be able to deliver timely immunizations for young children, Nurr'araaluk Davidson noted. The Community Health Aide Program was expanded into the Behavioral Health Aide Program, which focuses on mental health and substance abuse disorder treatment. The Dental Health Aide Therapist program is a mid-level dental program that provides dental services that were previously not offered and has helped children in Alaskan communities to become cavity free for the first time since contact. The federal Special Diabetes Program for Indians is also under way. Finally, she noted that improving the economic status of a community can be one of the most effective methods to improve the health of a community.

Alaska's tribal communities have been disproportionately affected by COVID-19, said Nurr'araaluk Davidson. These disparities can be

---

[6] Committee on Appropriations, House of Representatives, U.S. Congress. 2015. *Testimony of the Alaska Native Tribal Health Consortium*. 114th Cong., 1st Sess. March 25.

attributed to the effects of systemic and institutional racism on health status, health services funding, and access to care. COVID-19 in Alaska has largely been addressed through the Alaska Native Tribal Health Consortium, which has deployed rapid testing throughout Alaska, and by regional tribal health organizations that have taken the lead in Alaska's COVID-19 response.

RURAL DATA CHALLENGES IN THE HEALTHY PEOPLE 2020 INITIATIVE

Sirin Yaemsiri from the U.S. Government Accountability Office provided an overview of the Healthy People 2020 initiative with a focus on objectives that track data on rurality, and described some of the challenges encountered in tracking health data in rural areas.

Overview of the Healthy People Initiative

Yaemsiri explained that the Healthy People 2020 initiative is a national agenda that communicates a vision for improving health and achieving health equity,[7] as well as providing a framework for tracking the public health priorities of HHS.[8] The Healthy People 2020 initiative includes 1,150 specific, measurable objectives across 42 distinct topic areas with targets to be achieved over the 2010–2020 10-year period. She noted that a data tool has been developed to accompany this initiative.[9] The Healthy People 2030 initiative was released on August 18, 2020. An overarching goal of Healthy People 2020 has been to achieve health equity and eliminate disparities, including rural health disparities. For instance, one of the initiative's objectives is to increase the proportion of persons with medical insurance. Like all of the initiative's objectives, it has a defined baseline (i.e., 83.2 percent of persons had medical insurance in 2008), target proportion (100 percent), target-setting method (total coverage), and data sources used to track progress (the National Health Interview Survey, CDC, and the National Center for Health Statistics). The data tool provides access to tracking data for this objective. For instance, the data for health insurance coverage can be arranged nationally or by metro versus nonmetro areas

---

[7] Healthy People provides science-based national goals and objectives with 10-year targets designed to guide national health promotion and disease prevention efforts to improve the health of all people in the United States. More information about Healthy People is available at https://www.cdc.gov/nchs/healthy_people (accessed August 6, 2020).

[8] More information about the Healthy People initiative is available at https://www.healthypeople.gov (accessed July 7, 2020).

[9] More information about the Healthy People 2020 data tool is available at https://www.healthypeople.gov/2020/data-search (accessed August 3, 2020).

as defined by the Office of Management and Budget (OMB). She added that the initiative's various objectives are supported by more than 200 individual data systems, although not all of them are able to provide this level of granularity of data specific to rural areas. Of the more than 1,100 objectives in the Healthy People 2020 initiative, about one-third have rural data at the national level, but far fewer of the objectives have data from rural areas by state. Data systems that have state-level rural data include the National Vital Statistics System, the Behavioral Risk Factor Surveillance System, and the National Survey on Drug Use and Health.

Tracking Mortality in Urban and Rural Areas

Yaemsiri described how the National Vital Statistics System is used to track mortality in urban and rural areas related to cancer, COPD, coronary heart disease, diabetes, unintentional injury, stroke, and suicide (Talih and Huang, 2016; Yaemsiri et al., 2019). Age-adjusted rates for these seven causes of death are tracked by Healthy People 2020 objectives; rural and urban data for these objectives were disaggregated using OMB's 2013 county-based classification scheme. The age-adjusted death rates per 100,000 population in the United States between 2007 and 2017 were higher in rural areas than in urban areas for each of those seven causes of death (Yaemsiri et al., 2019). Additionally, none of the national targets for these seven causes of death had been achieved in rural populations by 2017. Among the seven mortality targets, four are getting worse in rural areas—mortality related to diabetes, COPD (45 years and older), unintentional injury, and suicide—while mortality attributable to coronary heart disease, cancer, and stroke are improving in rural areas (Yaemsiri et al., 2019). She noted that rural death rates are typically further from reaching national targets from the outset because objective targets are set based on national death rates, so rural areas have to make more progress to reach the targets. Yaemsiri suggested that these trends and the disparities in progress toward Healthy People 2020 targets between rural and urban areas is related to the notion of structural urbanism discussed by Janice Probst.

Challenges and Opportunities in Tracking Rural Health Data

Yaemsiri outlined some of the challenges encountered in efforts by the Heathy People 2020 initiative to track mortality in rural areas. Not all Healthy People data systems support estimates for rural areas at the national level, and far fewer support estimates for rural areas at the state level. Rural measures need to have at least two reliable and comparable estimates in order to measure progress toward national targets. As previously mentioned, targets are set based on national rates, often requiring rural areas to make greater progress than urban areas in order to meet those targets. The Healthy People data tool currently does not support estimates for rural areas by region, nor does it currently support aggregation of data years to improve the reliability of data in rural areas. Finally, the data tool lacks a feature that would allow researchers to easily filter and find objectives that have rural estimates at the national or state level.

She noted that an Agency for Healthcare Research and Quality (AHRQ) chart book on rural disparities has been released (AHRQ, 2017), along with a mid-course review of the Healthy People 2020 initiative (NCHS, 2016). For the Healthy People initiative to meet its overarching goal of reducing health disparities in rural areas, it will be necessary to track and measure progress for all rural areas, Yaemsiri said. Such tracking and measurement would allow for data users to flexibly aggregate data to produce reliable estimates for rural areas and for the creation of regional estimates for rural residents where it is not possible to make state estimates or to aggregate data years. Additionally, she suggested that data systems could do the following:

- Expand sample sizes to allow state estimates of Healthy People measures for rural residents.
- Oversample rural residents to allow for the creation of state estimates of Healthy People measures for rural residents.
- Allow implementers using custom data analyses to use Healthy People as a framework and benchmark for their data analyses.

RURAL HEALTHY PEOPLE INITIATIVE: PROCESSES AND RURAL HEALTH INDICATORS

Alva Ferdinand from the Southwest Rural Health Research Center at Texas A&M University discussed the development of the Rural Healthy People initiative, presented findings from Rural Healthy People surveys and publications, and described current and future plans to further advance the initiative's aims. Ferdinand explained that the Rural Healthy People initiative was commissioned by the Federal Office of Rural Health Policy in 2002 to complement HHS's Healthy People 2010 initiative. The aims of the Rural Healthy People initiative are to identify rural health priorities from the perspectives of various stakeholders and to consolidate those priorities with current research, practices, and models for addressing rural health priorities. She described efforts made by the initiative to date as well as plans for the future.

Rural Health Priorities Identified by the Rural Healthy People Initiative (2010 and 2020)

A major initial output of the Rural Healthy People initiative was the publication of *Rural Healthy People 2010*, a three-volume companion document to *Healthy People 2010* (Gamm et al., 2010) that identified and ranked the top 15 rural health priorities (see Table 3-1). After the successful dissemination of *Rural Healthy People 2010*, a Rural Healthy People 2020 advisory board was assembled in advance of Healthy People 2020, said Ferdinand. The advisory board included representatives from funding partners, rural health care providers, state rural health agencies, and national rural health agencies. The aims were to prioritize the objectives of the Healthy People initiative in terms of the needs of rural America and to engage with those working in the field to identify models and programs that were showing promise in rural settings. The advisory board developed a national survey to achieve these aims, with the findings from this survey to be disseminated to local, state, and federal policy makers. The board works with local, state, and federal agencies and other rural stakeholders to continue developing strategies for measurement and rural population health improvement.

The survey was first fielded in December 2010 with 755 respondents and again in Spring 2012 for a total of 1,214 respondents. Most states had 10 or more respondents, while 21 states had less than 10 respondents. Many of the survey respondents were health care administrators (31.7 percent), health care providers (26.8 percent), and health care educators (14.1 percent). The Rural Healthy People 2020 survey was used to identify the top 20 rural health priorities (see Figure 3-2). Ferdinand pointed out certain changes in rural health priorities between Rural Healthy People 2010 and Rural Healthy People 2020. Access to quality health care, diabetes, and mental health and mental disorders remained among the top five priorities. From 2010 to 2020, however, substance abuse and nutrition and weight status moved up in priority ranking among the top five priorities. Ferdinand noted that *Rural Healthy People 2020* was published in two volumes in 2015 (Bolin et al., 2015). The volumes were intended to address each of the rural health priorities and to identify innovative approaches that rural communities are using to meet Healthy People targets. Texas A&M University disseminated the *Rural Healthy People 2020* document from its website,[10] and the volumes have since been downloaded for many different purposes by a wide range of entities, including universities and colleges, hospitals, nonprofits, other health care clinics and

---

[10] The volumes are available at https://srhrc.tamhsc.edu/rhp2020/rhp2020-v1-download.html (accessed July 9, 2020) and https://srhrc.tamhsc.edu/rhp2020/rhp2020-v2-download.html (accessed July 9, 2020).

TABLE 3-1 Top Rural Health Priorities Identified by Rural Healthy People 2010 and Rural Healthy People 2020

	Rural Health Priority Objective	
Rank	Rural Healthy People 2010	Rural Healthy People 2020
1	Access to quality health care	Access to quality health care
2	Heart disease and stroke	Nutrition and weight status
3	Diabetes	Diabetes
4	Mental health and mental disorders	Mental health and mental disorders
5	Oral health	Substance abuse
6	Tobacco use	Heart disease and stroke
7	Substance abuse	Physical activity and health
8	Education and community-based programs	Older adults
9	Maternal, infant, and child health	Tobacco use
10	Nutrition and overweight status	Cancer
11	Public health infrastructure	Education and community-based programs
12	Immunization	Oral health
13	Injury and violence prevention	Quality of life and well-being
14	Family planning	Immunizations and infectious disease
15	Environmental health	Public health infrastructure
16	N/A	Family planning and sexual health
17	N/A	Injury and violence prevention
18	N/A	Social determinants of health
19	N/A	Health communication and health IT
20	N/A	Environmental health

NOTE: IT = information technology.
SOURCES: Adapted from Ferdinand presentation, June 24, 2020; Bolin et al., 2015; Gamm et al., 2010.

providers, state and municipal agencies, public health offices, and federal agencies, as well as volunteer and indigent clinics.

Rural Healthy People: Past, Present, and Future

Ferdinand highlighted some of the key features of the Rural Healthy People initiative thus far and described efforts under way for Rural Healthy People 2030. Rural Healthy People 2010 and Rural Healthy People 2020 shared certain key features. Both initiatives prioritized access to

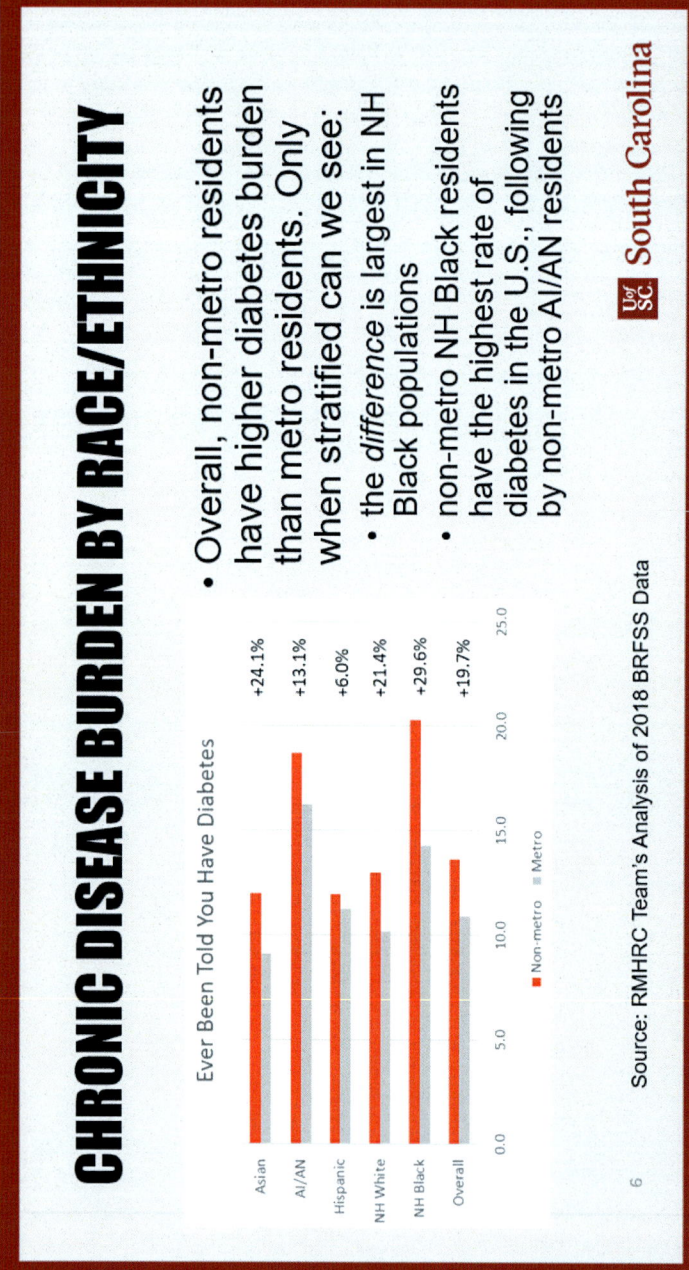

FIGURE 3-2 Chronic disease burden by race and ethnicity for diabetes.
NOTE: AI/AN = American Indian/Alaska Native; BRFSS = Behavioral and Risk Factor Surveillance System; NH = not Hispanic; RMHRC = (South Carolina) Rural and Minority Health Research Center.
SOURCE: Eberth presentation, June 24, 2020.

care as the highest-ranking rural health priority. She surmised that this is likely to remain the highest rural health priority going forward, especially as the COVID-19 pandemic unfolds and continues to impact rural communities. Both iterations of Rural Healthy People reflected a great need for additional model programs and practices that have been shown to be effective in rural settings, along with the need for new targeted prevention and care models for rural areas.

Rural Healthy People 2030 will continue to seek the input and involvement of rural stakeholders, with the following aims:

- identifying objectives within priority areas for targeted attention between 2020 and 2030,
- identifying successful or promising programs developed in rural America that will help achieve those objectives,
- identifying and advocating for data sources that will help track the progress of rural America toward Healthy People targets, and
- keeping rural health disparities at the forefront of policy makers' and advocates' minds.

She added that the Rural Healthy People 2030 initiative has experienced delays because the Healthy People 2030 release was hindered by the COVID-19 pandemic. Nevertheless, the Rural Healthy People 2030 project is expected to once again help bring together researchers and practitioners to identify the rural health issues that demand the greatest attention in the coming years.

THE EFFECT OF RACIAL DISPARITIES IN RURAL AREAS

Jan Eberth from the Rural and Minority Health Research Center at the University of South Carolina considered how racial and ethnic disparities may be lost in the broader discussion of rural–urban disparities. She contextualized health equity in rural settings; discussed the intersection of race, ethnicity, and mortality in the COVID-19 pandemic; and concluded by considering the implications of racial and ethnic disparities in the rural context.

Health Inequity in the Rural Context

Noting that rural America is economically, socially, and demographically diverse, Eberth examined how the discrete differences in health across the rural–urban spectrum can mask substantial differences across racial and ethnic lines. She defined race as a socially defined classification that exposes some individuals to interpersonal and structural disadvantages. In rural America, one in five persons is a person of color or an Indigenous person. Metro populations are more diverse, with about 42 percent racial or ethnic minorities, and most of the growth in nonmetro areas in the past two decades can be attributed to nonwhite persons. In particular, the Hispanic population is growing in rural areas by approximately 2 percent per year on average (Cromartie, 2018).

Mortality is one of the most basic measures of population health, but Eberth noted that mortality data aggregated across rural areas can mask key differences in the experiences of people living within those rural communities. Between 1999 and 2017, age-adjusted all-cause mortality rates per 100,000 remained relatively steady for nonmetro non-Hispanic white populations, declining at a rate of 0.34 percent per year on average (Probst et al., 2020).[11] During the same period, American Indian, Alaska Native, and Black populations living in nonmetro areas had reductions in all-cause mortality averaging 0.52 percent per year for American Indian and Alaska Native populations, and 1.04 percent per year for nonmetro African American populations. However, although the all-cause mortality rates decreased, the absolute mortality rate remained higher than that of non-Hispanic white populations. The most prominent reductions in all-cause mortality during the period were observed among nonmetro Asian and Pacific Islander populations (2.46 percent average reduction per year) and among nonmetro Hispanic populations (1.85 percent average reduction per year). Eberth added that both groups have consistently maintained lower absolute all-cause mortality rates than their nonmetro white peers. She pointed out that since 2009, nonmetro mortality rates across all races and ethnicities have nearly leveled off and increased slightly among some groups, but most of the declines were observed in the early 2000s.

The leading causes of death in the United States are cancer, cardiovascular disease, and unintentional injury. According to CDC data, from 2013 to 2017, nonmetro residents experienced higher age-adjusted death rates than their urban peers for all three causes of death, with disparities of 13 percent in cancer mortality, 20 percent in cardiovascular disease mortality, and 37 percent in mortality caused by unintentional injury (Probst et al., 2020). Regardless of metro/nonmetro designation, Asian and Pacific Islander populations have the lowest mortality rates for all three of these causes of death, Black populations have the highest rates of mortality caused by cancer and cardiovascular disease, and American Indian and Alaska Native populations have the highest rates of mortality caused by unintentional injuries. Notably, the largest gap between

---

[11] More information about CDC's Wide-ranging Online Data for Epidemiologic Research (WONDER) online databases is available at https://wonder.cdc.gov/controller/datarequest/D76 (accessed August 6, 2020).

metro and nonmetro populations within a single racial or ethnic group is found in American Indian and Alaska Native populations. Among this group, nonmetro residents had a rate of mortality attributable to cancer and cardiovascular disease that was 33 percent higher than that for urban residents and a rate of death attributable to unintentional injury that was 60 percent higher than that for urban residents.

Eberth presented data on infant mortality rates between 2015 and 2017 for metro and nonmetro populations stratified by race and ethnicity to demonstrate the high rates of infant mortality among both metro and nonmetro Black populations—about 11 per 1,000 persons in both metro and nonmetro populations—and to highlight the 82 percent disparity between metro and nonmetro American Indian and Alaska Native populations (5.5 and 10 per 1,000 in metro versus nonmetro populations, respectively) (Probst et al., 2019). She added that similar data showing racial and ethnic differences and childhood mortality can be found in the *Health Affairs* 2019 special issue on rural health.[12]

Eberth noted that in addition to mortality, morbidity is also a key indicator of population health that often differs by race and ethnicity in metro versus nonmetro populations. For instance, according to 2018 data on the proportions of metro and nonmetro populations who report having been diagnosed with diabetes, nonmetro populations had a greater diabetes burden than metro populations within each racial and ethnic designation.[13] Stratifying these data by race shows that the metro versus nonmetro gap in diabetes diagnosis is greatest among non-Hispanic Black populations. Overall, nonmetro non-Hispanic Black populations have the highest rate of diabetes in the United States, followed by nonmetro American Indian and Alaska Native populations (see Figure 3-2).

Nonmetro populations were also more likely than metro populations to have ever been diagnosed with COPD or cancer.[14] With the exception of nonmetro American Indian and Alaska Native populations, all other nonmetro racial and ethnic groups were more likely than their metro peers to have been diagnosed with COPD or cancer, she added.

---

[12] More information about the *Health Affairs* 2019 special issue on rural health is available at https://www.healthaffairs.org/toc/hlthaff/38/12 (accessed July 10, 2020).

[13] These data were collected from the CDC Behavioral Risk Factor Surveillance System Survey and analyzed by the Rural and Minority Health Research Center at the University of South Carolina. More information about the CDC Behavioral Risk Factor Surveillance System Survey is available at https://www.cdc.gov/brfss/annual_data/annual_2018.html (accessed July 10, 2020).

[14] More information is available at https://www.cdc.gov/copd/features/copd-urban-rural-differences.html (accessed August 6, 2020).

COVID-19, Race, and Ethnicity

Eberth discussed the intersection of mortality, race, and ethnicity in the COVID-19 pandemic. One study based on data from early 2020 through mid-April 2020 found that 52 percent of COVID-19 cases and nearly 60 percent of COVID-19 deaths occurred in counties with a disproportionately high proportion of Black residents (Millett et al., 2020). The researchers stratified COVID-19 rates by urbanicity and found that the relationship between COVID-19 diagnoses and having a high proportion of Black residents was similar across all levels of urbanicity. However, the risk of COVID-19 death that was associated with a higher proportion of Black residents was only significant in small metropolitan and noncore areas. She added that 91 percent of these disproportionately Black counties are located in the American South, which is the region where the majority of Black Americans live. The study also found that a COVID-19 diagnosis was independently associated with the percentage of uninsured residents. She noted that it will be necessary to follow up on these findings to determine whether these trends persist, worsen, or improve as the pandemic continues, particularly as the number of COVID-19 cases continues to rise throughout the American South.

Root Causes of Health Inequity in Rural Areas

Eberth explained that for traditionally underserved populations, living in a rural area can "heighten exposure to unequal social conditions that perpetuate disparities" (Caldwell et al., 2016). The root causes of health inequity in rural areas include higher rates of poverty, lower educational attainment, lower access to health care services, failing infrastructure and lower per capita investment, lack of public transportation, and segregation and racism. She noted that both compositional and contextual factors related to SDOH[15] may also mediate or modify observed racial or ethnic differences in health outcomes (Lorch and Enlow, 2016). Compositional factors, such as median income in an area, reflect underlying characteristics of the people who live in those areas. Contextual factors represent area-level properties that are often modifiable and not directly linked to the characteristics of the people who live in an area. Common examples of contextual factors include zoning laws for affordable housing and state-level policies that dictate Medicaid qualification criteria.

The prevalence of certain SDOH varies by race and ethnicity among rural residents, she added (Probst et al., 2019). Rural residents who are Black, Hispanic, and American Indian or Alaska Native are more likely

---

[15] The SDOH include neighborhoods and the built environment, health and health care, social and community context, education, and economic stability.

to be living in poverty, have attained less than a high school education, and are more likely to be without broadband than rural residents who are white or Asian. Rural Black and American Indian and Alaska Native populations have the greatest rates of poverty and the least access to broadband. Eberth noted that this is a critical concern in light of the response to the COVID-19 pandemic, which has relied heavily on the implementation of online schooling and telehealth. A large proportion of rural Hispanic residents have less than a high school education. Hispanic populations were also least likely to report having any health care coverage in the 2008 CDC Behavioral Risk Factor Surveillance System Survey.[16]

Addressing the Compounding Effects of Rurality and Racial and Ethnic Minority Status

Eberth emphasized the compounding effects of rurality and racial and ethnic minority status on health. In rural areas, racial and ethnic minorities experience higher rates of mortality across the life span, have higher rates of chronic disease in adulthood, and are more likely to experience adverse social and economic conditions. Together, these factors can contribute to, create, and exacerbate health inequalities. Given the effects of rurality on ethnic and minority groups, Eberth asserted that interventions aimed at addressing inequality must be designed with a focus on rural populations. Most existing interventions that target inequity rely on mechanisms of behavior change and require buy-in at the individual level. However, population-level interventions that do not require high levels of individual agency—though less common than individual-level interventions—have been shown to be more effective (Frieden, 2010). She maintained that policies should be developed and enforced to ensure equitable education, housing, health care, transportation, and criminal justice that are "right sized" for rural settings. To successfully effect real improvement in rural health, she added, policies should focus on SDOH and macro-level factors across multiple sectors beyond an exclusive focus on the health care system.

DISCUSSION

Disseminating Rural Health Data to Rural Communities

Knudson started the discussion and asked how to best distribute data to rural communities so they can address their own local issues. Holmes

---

[16] More information about the CDC Behavioral Risk Factor Surveillance System Survey is available at https://www.cdc.gov/brfss/annual_data/annual_2008.htm (accessed July 10, 2020).

acknowledged CDC's progress in making its data rural friendly, especially through the development of the CDC Wide-ranging Online Data for Epidemiologic Research online databases and its implementation of a metro/nonmetro indicator.[17] Other entities have also made efforts to disseminate and aid in the dissemination of rural health data, he added, so new approaches for increasing publications and building awareness of such efforts would be beneficial.

Nurr'araaluk Davidson commented on the need for buy-in from communities where data are being collected. She noted that in Alaska, researchers are struggling with a historical legacy of misappropriation of data collected from tribal communities. For instance, she mentioned that states or other implementers often use data from tribal communities, which frequently reveal poor health outcomes, to apply for grants that are not used to serve those communities. Good stewardship and a spirit of partnership are critical for using community data appropriately, she said. Alaska benefits from Alaskan Epicenter, a tribally operated epidemiology center at the Alaska Native Tribal Health Consortium that is 1 of 12 national epicenters that are either operated by tribes themselves or by IHS. She emphasized that in keeping with the adage "nothing about us without us," tribal communities should be the primary beneficiaries of data collected from them.

Ferdinand added that researchers who collect data often make paternalistic assumptions about the people whose data they collect without engaging with them to find out how they would like their data to be used. For instance, people with chronic diseases might be more willing to allow their data to be used if the data can contribute to improvements in population health. Rather than starting with whatever data are already available, she suggested that researchers should ask populations for input about what types of data to collect and how they would be comfortable with those data being used (e.g., linking data across hospitals or other data enterprises).

Yaemsiri suggested that data systems should oversample from rural areas in order to provide better estimates of rural health. Existing data resources should also be used in more flexible ways in order to present rural health estimates at the regional level or aggregate data by year, which can be used to evaluate progress in rural areas over time. She noted that in addition to rural populations, these strategies can benefit small population groups—such as the Native Hawaiian and other Pacific Islander, American Indian, and Alaska Native populations—for which obtaining reliable data may require aggregating over geographic areas or

---

[17] More information about CDC WONDER online databases is available at https://wonder.cdc.gov (accessed July 9, 2020).

data years. She added that the forthcoming Healthy People 2030 initiative will include far fewer objectives than Healthy People 2020, allowing for a greater focus on smaller subpopulations within each objective. Eberth added that much of the data on SDOH come from the U.S. Census. Proposed changes for the U.S. Census include additional privacy rules and the introduction of "noise" in Census data for small areas, which could have the unintended consequence of inhibiting the quality of data collected from small populations.

The Effect of Barriers to Accessing Care in Rural Communities

A participant asked whether there are significantly higher death rates for diabetes and cancer in rural areas due to higher prevalence and complications caused by systemic lack of access to care, treatment, or follow-up. Eberth replied that people with cancer in rural areas face greater barriers to accessing specialists, like oncologists, gastroenterologists, and cancer surgeons, which may require traveling long distances from their homes. Holmes noted that along the care trajectory, small gaps of just 5 percent can have cumulative and compounding effects in terms of delays in timely diagnoses, follow-up, and treatment. Nurr'araaluk Davidson added that in tribal communities throughout the country, the shift away from their traditional diets has contributed greatly to population health challenges. They have also observed correlations between adverse childhood experiences and health status in tribal communities. She noted that the Special Diabetes Program for Indians has brought about substantial improvements because the program offers latitude for tribes and tribal health organizations to tailor diabetes programs to the needs of local populations with services such as nutrition classes, ensuring that fresh vegetables are available, and encouraging residents to harvest natural foods.

Social Determinants of Health Within the Healthy People Initiative

Given that the SDOH account for at least 40 percent of health outcomes, a participant asked why the SDOH are not a top priority within the Healthy People initiative. Yaemsiri explained that measures of the SDOH are accounted for in each objective in the Healthy People 2020 initiative in that under the national tracking data, the initiative also tracks data by race and ethnicity, education, income, geographic location by state, and other factors that help measure the SDOH. Additionally, the initiative includes an SDOH topic area with cross-cutting objectives. She suggested that addressing the SODH more effectively will require a national shift in focus away from national rates and toward the underlying social determinants. Ferdinand commented that the Rural Healthy People initiative may have missed an opportunity to highlight the SDOH more prominently, but the effects of those determinants on health outcomes are being increasingly articulated and considered in rural health contexts. Subsequent iterations of Rural Healthy People will have the opportunity to unpack the SDOH and engage with stakeholders to determine where they fall in priority among rural health priorities, she added.

Acceleration of Telehealth in Response to COVID-19: Implications for Rural Health

Probst asked whether the transition to telehealth accelerated by the COVID-19 pandemic has served as an effective mechanism for improving infrastructure for rural areas. Holmes commented that the promise of telehealth is still undermined by the lack of Internet bandwidth and broadband capacity. However, the pandemic circumstances have demonstrated that an aggressive and accelerated transition toward expanded telehealth services can be executed with relative success in terms of convenience and quality, depending on the service being delivered. Holmes suggested that in addition to expediting the process of embracing telehealth more broadly, this aggressive shift may also help to equalize the rural–urban gap in health care access, but this only applies to rural residents with high-speed Internet connectivity in the privacy of their own homes, which many do not have. In that respect, much work remains to be done to improve telehealth from both equity and operational standpoints, he added.

Nurr'araaluk Davidson remarked that the expansion of patient-centered telehealth opportunities in response to the COVID-19 pandemic was long overdue, and it has been helpful in refuting the conventional wisdom that telehealth is inefficient, ineffective, and precluded by bandwidth limitations. Telehealth through the Alaska Federal Health Care Access Network has been in use for years and has been transformative in offering rural residents access to higher-quality health care services as well as substantial savings in the high costs of travel to access health care services of any kind from many rural communities.[18] To address bandwidth

---

[18] Rural residents often must pay $1,000 to fly to the nearest health care provider, which is unsustainable for many families, given that the typical annual family income for a rural family may be as low as $20,000.

issues in rural Alaska, people can now visit many village health clinics to access telehealth services from providers that would otherwise be inaccessible. Eberth added that the COVID-19 pandemic has also brought about positive regulatory changes, with certain long-standing rules loosened to facilitate the rapid acceleration of telehealth. For instance, telephone visits, which have traditionally been disallowed, are being used to circumvent broadband issues in some communities that have better access to telephone services than Internet services. She suggested that it could be beneficial to make some of these regulatory changes more permanent going forward.

4

Rural Health Care in Action

The third session of the workshop focused on the national landscape of rural health care services, the role of tribal health care entities across rural America, the function of wraparound services in rural communities, and the contribution of community health workers (CHWs) to rural health care. The session was moderated by Tom Morris from the Federal Office of Rural Health Policy at the Health Resources and Services Administration (HRSA).

RURAL HEALTH CARE LANDSCAPE

Paul Moore from the Federal Office of Rural Health Policy at HRSA presented data on rural health provider infrastructure, explored challenges and disparities in rural health care, and discussed the impact of the coronavirus disease 2019 (COVID-19) on health care access in rural communities. He remarked that although fewer doctors in rural areas are making house calls and delivering babies in local emergency departments (EDs) than in the past, independent physicians in rural towns continue to feature prominently in the rural health care landscape (e.g., by staffing EDs as needed and making hospital rounds on their patients before they begin their in-office practice each day).

The Rural Health Care Safety Net

Moore explained that rural health care infrastructure largely comprises small hospitals and clinics that have special reimbursement terms from the key public payers—Medicare and Medicaid. These public programs designate three types of providers in rural areas: critical access hospitals (CAHs), rural health clinics, and federally qualified health centers (FQHCs). Together, these types of care providers compose "the rural health safety net."

Moore provided more detail on these three types of provider designations. CAHs were created as a special designation under Medicare by the Balanced Budget Act of 1997. These facilities have a limit of 25 beds or less and a limitation on length of stay, which currently averages 96 hours.[1] Of the approximately 2,000 rural hospitals nationwide, more than 1,450 are CAHs. He added that in most rural communities, small rural hospitals and CAHs often serve as the linchpin of the health care system. Although a substantial number of local, county, or city-owned and managed hospitals are still in operation, system consolidation is on the rise. This is leading to a mix of systems in some settings, such as urban health systems that include some rural providers, mixed rural and urban systems, and private management affiliations and groups of hospitals. The designation "rural health clinic" was created in 1977 as part of the Rural Health Clinic Services Act.[2] Rural health clinics receive certification from the Centers for Medicare & Medicaid Services (CMS) based in part on their location. These clinics, which receive special all-inclusive rate payments, can be either independent or provider based and must be staffed by both physicians and either nurse practitioners or physician assistants.

FQHCs are administered by HRSA's Bureau of Primary Healthcare after being established in the 1960s as part of the war on poverty.[3] Designed as a demonstration program to provide access to health and social services to medically underserved and disenfranchised populations, FQHCs are located in both urban and rural areas. Currently, about 40 percent of the 14,000 FQHC sites are in rural communities. FQHCs provide a menu of services and are required to see all patients regardless of ability to pay, he noted.

---

[1] More information about the critical access hospital designation is available at https://www.cms.gov/Outreach-and-Education/Medicare-Learning-Network-MLN/MLNProducts/Downloads/CritAccessHospfctsht.pdf (accessed July 30, 2020).

[2] More information about the rural health clinic designation is available at https://www.cms.gov/Outreach-and-Education/Medicare-Learning-Network-MLN/MLNProducts/Downloads/RuralHlthClinfctsht.pdf (accessed July 30, 2020).

[3] More information about the FQHC designation is available at https://www.cms.gov/Outreach-and-Education/Medicare-Learning-Network-MLN/MLNProducts/Downloads/fqhcfactsheet.pdf (accessed July 30, 2020).

These three types of designated providers are examples of how various federal policy levers, such as reimbursement, are used to support rural hospitals, clinics, and providers, said Moore. However, many other types of providers play important roles in the rural health care landscape. These include long-term care facilities that serve Medicare and dual-eligible Medicaid patient populations, nursing homes, assisted living facilities, and residential services for people with disabilities.[4] Other types of rural service providers include tribal clinics and hospitals, Veterans Affairs clinics and hospitals, home health care, hospice, occupational therapy, speech therapy, physical therapy, pharmacies, dentists, mental and behavioral health providers, and community health aides.

Disparities in the Rural Health Care Landscape

Moore outlined various disparities in the rural health care landscape. He remarked that despite the broad range of health care facilities and providers who serve rural areas, maldistribution within the health care workforce infrastructure is a major issue. While approximately 18 percent of the nation's population is rural, only 10 percent of primary care practitioners and less than 7 percent of specialty care practitioners reside in rural areas. Furthermore, approximately 5 percent of rural counties do not have any family physicians.

The negative effects on rural health care are evident across what Moore describes as the "five Ds": death rates, disparities, distance, dollars, and departures. *Death rates* show that the life expectancy in rural areas is 3 years shorter than for people in urban areas. Furthermore, rural communities have higher death rates for heart disease and stroke. Rural women face higher maternal mortality rates than their urban counterparts. *Disparities* are present in a number of health factors, in part because rural residents face higher rates of tobacco use, physical inactivity, obesity, diabetes, and high blood pressure. The disparity in the distribution of and access to health care providers extends beyond physical health care, he added. Rural populations face greater challenges with mental and behavioral health than people living in urban areas, yet they generally have limited access to mental health care. *Distance* is also a factor, given that rural areas have limited or nonexistent public transportation infrastructure. Rural residents often face long distances between their homes and health care providers and do not always have access to a vehicle, making it difficult to access emergency care, specialty care, and preventive care.

---

[4] More information about long-term care facilities is available at https://www.ruralhealthinfo.org/topics/long-term-care (accessed July 30, 2020).

He explained that *dollars* pertains to the economics of rural areas, as rural populations are more likely to be uninsured or underinsured and typically have fewer affordable health insurance options than their urban counterparts. *Departure* refers to the closure of rural health care facilities: since January 2010, 130 rural hospitals have closed (Thomas et al., 2019). Of these, 43 were CAHs receiving cost-based Medicare reimbursement, which indicates that these CAHs were so financially vulnerable that this reimbursement was not sufficient to keep them open. The remaining 87 hospitals were noncritical access or prospective payment system hospitals with other Medicare designations. He added that many more rural hospitals are continuing to operate with a high degree of financial vulnerability.

Innovations in the Rural Health Care Landscape

Moore also described some of the innovations that are taking place in the rural health landscape to counteract some of the negative trends. Successful examples that can provide helpful insights include the Frontier Extended Stay Clinic, the recently closed Frontier Community Health Integration project, the Rural Community Hospital Demonstration program, and rural state innovation models.[5] CMS has ongoing rural value-based initiatives such as accountable care organizations (ACOs), which are making good inroads in rural areas. The next generation of the ACO model includes state-located models, such as Vermont's all-payer ACO system as well as the Pennsylvania rural health model.[6] He noted that the latter model uses global budgeting, and thus far, hospitals with global budgets appear more resistant to pandemic-induced fluctuations caused by the cancellation of elective surgeries and outpatient appointments.

Impact of COVID-19 in Rural Areas

The COVID-19 pandemic has created new challenges and opportunities in rural areas, said Moore. The increasing COVID-19 case numbers in rural states appear to dispel the idea that rural communities with more space might fare better than urban areas. He noted that rural regions such as western Kansas and Oklahoma did not initially see the COVID-19 transmission rates that urban centers such as New York City and Chicago experienced, but those rural areas were experiencing a dramatic

---

[5] More information about rural health models and innovations is available at https://www.ruralhealthinfo.org/project-examples (accessed July 30, 2020).

[6] More information about the Pennsylvania Rural Health Model is available at https://innovation.cms.gov/innovation-models/pa-rural-health-model (accessed July 30, 2020).

increase in cases as of late June 2020.[7] He remarked that the pandemic has shone a glaring light on enduring and far-reaching issues, including the racial, ethnic, and economic health disparities in rural areas, and it has underscored the need to improve access and surge capacity in rural areas. He suggested that there are opportunities associated with COVID-19 as well, given that "a few months of pandemic accomplished in telehealth what years of advocacy could not." Moore also proposed that alternative payment models and system designs may better align with the need to maintain access to quality health care services in the rural health care landscape than the current structures.

TRIBAL HEALTH AND HEALTH CARE IN RURAL SETTINGS

Daniel Calac from the Indian Health Council discussed the diversity among American Indian populations, the magnitude of American Indian/Alaska Native health disparities, the factors affecting the quality of life, and the severity of the biomedical workforce shortage affecting this sector of the U.S. population. The American Indian presence in the United States is highly diverse. Nearly 600 tribes currently live across the country, with more than 570 of these officially recognized by the U.S. federal government.[8] Language varies between tribes, as indicated by the existence of more than 350 distinct dialects. Furthermore, native individuals may have distinct customs and diverse cultural norms that contribute to the level of care they deem appropriate. Substantial variety may exist even among nearby tribes, he added. For example, Calac's organization near San Diego County serves nine individual reservations and tribes that are located within a 5-mile radius, all of which have their own unique customs.

Historical Context for the Provision of Health Care to American Indians

Calac provided some historical perspective about the lingering impact of colonialism and past treaties with the U.S. government on the way many tribal entities perceive health care. As part of negotiations between American Indian nations and the U.S. government, a prepaid health care plan was pledged for native people. However, a common sentiment is that this health plan was prepaid by the cession of the entirety of the

---

[7] More information about rural and urban COVID-19 hotspots is available at https://www.shepscenter.unc.edu/programs-projects/rural-health/rural-covid-research-and-figures/rural-and-urban-covid-19-hot-spots (accessed July 30, 2020).

[8] See https://www.ncsl.org/research/state-tribal-institute/list-of-federal-and-state-recognized-tribes.aspx (accessed October 28, 2020).

American Indian peoples' lands (Rhoades and Derre Smith, 1996). This perception is compounded by a rural health care system that is struggling to maintain an adequate level of increasingly complex care for American Indian populations.

When American Indians traded land with fertile soil or river access to the United States, the treaty obligations and the needs of this population did not evaporate with their relocation, said Calac. The U.S. government has shifted responsibility for meeting these obligations to various agencies over time. Initially, a division within the Department of War oversaw health services for American Indians. In 1849, this responsibility was transferred to the Bureau of Indian Affairs. Congress ratified appropriations with the 1921 Snyder Act, landmark legislation that defined the governmental responsibility for American Indian health care. Service delivery for American Indians was transferred to the Public Health Service in 1954 before shifting again to the newly formed Indian Health Service (IHS) the following year (Warne and Frizzell, 2014). The Indian Health Care Improvement Act of 1976 was another landmark piece of legislation, which offered assurances for the delivery of high-quality health care for the underserved Indigenous population.

Indian Health Service in the 21st Century

Calac explained that IHS currently has 12 service areas across the United States. Regardless of geography or the specific tribal entities, the burden of disease and health care disparities are common throughout these service areas.[9] IHS operates 31 hospitals and 50 health centers, some of which are FQHCs. Two school-based IHS health centers enable service delivery to at-risk children, including the preventive health care needed at younger ages. IHS also oversees 31 health stations that were developed collaboratively by individual tribes and the IHS over the past 50 to 60 years. Calac said these stations offer more appropriate care than settings serving larger populations, because they provide an individualized level of care tailored to the communities they serve. Given the differences among the 570 distinct tribes, this type of community-specific approach is critical for meeting the specific needs of tribal entities.

Many Indian health care clinics rely on grant funding to provide basic health care to tribal communities. Calac's organization, the Indian Health Council, uses a facility model that has been replicated throughout California, a state that is home to 42 Indian health care clinics and 7 urban Indian health clinics. This type of facility offers a multidisciplinary range

---

[9] More information about IHS areas and locations is available at https://www.ihs.gov/locations (accessed July 30, 2020).

of services, such as medical, dental, and medical subspecialties, including optometry, acupuncture, and behavioral health; these facilities also address public health issues affecting tribal entities. He added that this approach to a clinic as a "health village" rather than a "health facility" helps to engage people and imbue them with a sense of ownership of the clinics, thus encouraging people to access services.

Health Disparities for American Indians and Alaska Natives

American Indians and Alaska Natives experience many health disparities, said Calac. Determinants of health equity include

- limitations in communication capacity and resources,
- variability in health literacy,
- lack of community engagement and awareness,
- limited financial resources,
- transportation challenges,
- displacement effects,
- variability in implementation,
- crime and safety influences (real and perceived), and
- lack of awareness of diverse norms and customs.[10]

He noted that health literacy is a fundamental component of health equity that is particularly relevant in the context of the COVID-19 pandemic, such as understanding the difference between an antibody test and a polymerase chain reaction test, knowing what RNA means in terms of viral particles, and knowing the appropriate doses of over-the-counter medications, such as acetaminophen. Transportation is an aspect of health equity that is particularly relevant for rural communities, he noted. Multiple challenges come into play when people in rural areas have long distances between their homes and health care, such as adequate infrastructure in terms of roads and access to vehicles. Finally, crime and safety influences on health equity can be seen in the opioid epidemic, which is heavily affecting rural areas. Calac added that challenges related to Mexican cartels trafficking heroin through rural areas, as well as human trafficking in these regions, are also continuing problems. These types of disparities in health equity result in disparities in measures such as life expectancy, he emphasized. The life span of American Indians, at a

---

[10] More information about the Centers for Disease Control and Prevention guidelines for advancing health equity and preventing chronic disease is available at https://www.cdc.gov/nccdphp/dnpao/state-local-programs/health-equity-guide/index.htm (accessed July 30, 2020).

median 76 years, is 5 years shorter than the median 81 years of the general population. Calac stated that in more impoverished areas, such as in the Dakotas, and in areas distant from hospitals and major clinics, the average life span can be as much as 20 years shorter for some native populations.

Factors Affecting the Quality of Life of Tribal Communities

Calac highlighted some of the many factors that affect the quality of life of American Indians and Alaska Natives, including barriers to accessing health care that are geographic, educational, institutional, social, or financial. Distance to health care providers can be a geographic barrier to care, as can mountainous regions that are difficult and even dangerous to traverse. Educational barriers are evidenced by lower graduation rates. In 2014–2015, the American Indian population had a high school graduation rate of 71.6 percent, compared to 83.2 percent for the general population. This disparity is even greater at the postsecondary level, with 19.8 percent of American Indians receiving a bachelor's degree versus 32.5 percent of all adults in the United States.[11] Institutional challenges include the funding cycle for IHS, which is year to year instead of the protracted 5-year or 10-year budget cycle that corporations and many communities can rely on for funding individual programs. Furthermore, IHS programs are consistently underfunded by as much as 40 percent, with prominent shortages in funding for mental health. Calac said a social barrier is the ongoing and persistent trend of low use of preventive health care due to the perception of health care as the use of urgent or emergency care. Lastly, the financial barriers faced by the American Indian population are substantial. In 2014, approximately 28 percent of the Indigenous population was living in poverty compared with 15.5 percent for all Americans.[12] Per capita health care spending on American Indians is also lower than for other populations. In 2005, IHS spent an average of $3,099 per recipient, less than half of the $8,097 per capita rate for Medicaid recipients.[13] Calac added that this disparity has not changed much since 2005, with IHS receiving lower per capita medical expense rates than even the Federal Bureau of Prisons.

---

[11] More information about rates of high school completion and bachelor's degree attainment among persons age 25 and over by race/ethnicity and sex is available at https://nces.ed.gov/programs/digest/d15/tables/dt15_104.10.asp?current=yes (accessed July 30, 2020).

[12] More information about poverty rates among American Indian and Native American populations is available at https://www.census.gov/newsroom/facts-for-features/2015/cb15-ff22.html (accessed July 30, 2020).

[13] More information is available at https://www.aamc.org/news-insights/more-native-american-doctors-needed-reduce-health-disparities-their-communities (accessed July 30, 2020).

Calac noted the IHS health care workforce shortage across all types of health care providers. In 2015, IHS had vacancy rates of 16 percent for pharmacists, 24 percent for nurses, 26 percent for dentists, 32 percent for physician assistants, 34 percent for physicians, and 35 percent for advanced practice registered nurses. Furthermore, the matriculation rates of American Indian medical students are low. According to the Association of American Medical Colleges' 2017 data for medical school graduates, of the 93,000 individuals who graduated between 2012 and 2017, only 131 identified as American Indian or Alaska Native—a number of graduates that is insufficient to meet the needs of 570 different tribal entities. Calac emphasized that this and the underfunding of IHS pose major problems for the delivery of health care and the improvement of health care in these populations.

WRAPAROUND SERVICES: IMPLICATIONS FOR RURAL AMERICA

Nir Menachemi from Indiana University provided an overview of wraparound services, wraparound program outcomes, challenges to the adoption of this service delivery model, and implications for rural health. He noted that although the majority of studies he presented were conducted in urban areas—mostly in FQHCs in inner-city urban areas—these types of wraparound services would also benefit rural areas.

Overview of Wraparound Services

Menachemi explained that the term *wraparound* applies to nonmedical services provided in conjunction with primary care. Traditional wraparound services include social work, behavioral health, nutrition and diet, pharmacy assistance, and patient navigation. More recently, wraparound services have included financial counseling, which assists individuals in managing nonmedical aspects of their lives to enable them to better manage medical issues. Similarly, medical–legal partnerships have formed because legal services addressing challenges in people's lives may increase their ability to focus on and maintain health. Traditionally, access to these types of services has been via referrals to outside agencies. However, some FQHCs are now collocating these services with primary care and scheduling wraparound service providers to meet with patients at their primary care appointments, thereby increasing use of these services.

Most wraparound services are designed to address one or more of the social determinants of health (SDOH), said Menachemi. Figure 4-1 depicts wraparound services related to each SDOH and the health outcomes associated with those SDOH. For example, social workers can assist with

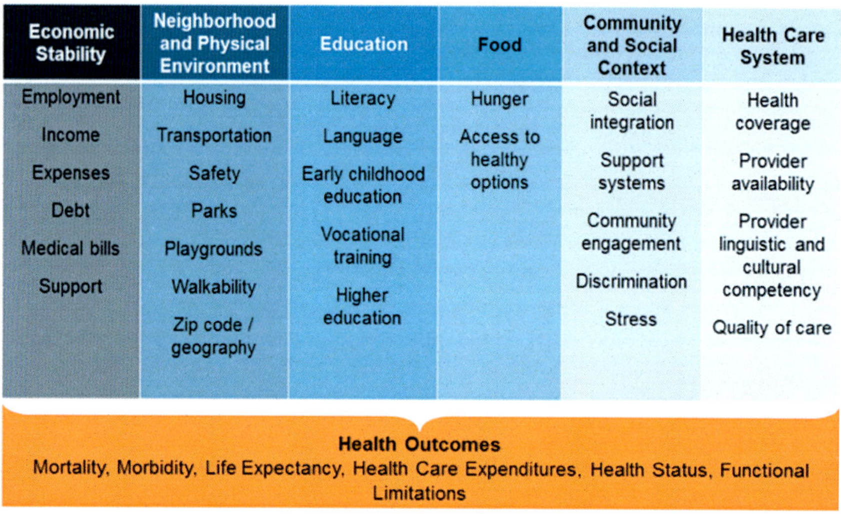

Economic Stability	Neighborhood and Physical Environment	Education	Food	Community and Social Context	Health Care System
Employment	Housing	Literacy	Hunger	Social integration	Health coverage
Income	Transportation	Language	Access to healthy options	Support systems	Provider availability
Expenses	Safety	Early childhood education		Community engagement	Provider linguistic and cultural competency
Debt	Parks	Vocational training		Discrimination	
Medical bills	Playgrounds			Stress	Quality of care
Support	Walkability	Higher education			
	Zip code / geography				

Health Outcomes
Mortality, Morbidity, Life Expectancy, Health Care Expenditures, Health Status, Functional Limitations

FIGURE 4-1 Wraparound services to address social determinants of health.
SOURCES: Menachemi presentation, June 24, 2020; https://www.kff.org/disparities-policy/issue-brief/beyond-health-care-the-role-of-social-determinants-in-promoting-health-and-health-equity (accessed August 5, 2020).

vocational training or housing issues, and dieticians focus on matters related to food and nutrition. Mental health counselors can help people provide information to manage stress and, to some degree, cope with discrimination, address social integration, and support systems. Wraparound services can include anything that enhances an individual's ability to maintain health or cope with disease, he added, because wraparound service providers are essentially working to mitigate the potentially negative effects of certain SDOH.

Wraparound Program Outcomes

A number of studies have measured the effect of wraparound services on patient outcomes, said Menachemi. In one study, referrals by health care professionals to social service providers led to a decrease in patient-reported needs, indicating that social services were able to address and eliminate some patient needs (Gottlieb et al., 2016). Wraparound services also increased parent and caregiver perception that their children's health needs were being met. Another study examined medical–legal wraparound partnerships in which attorneys provide pro bono consultative services to people in health care settings; it found these partnerships address legal issues that exacerbate poor health (Sandel et al., 2010). An example of how medical–legal partnerships can address such issues is the addition of legal forms to electronic health records, which can aid in processes such as rectifying substandard housing conditions for low-income patients. Other cases might involve a parent who is unable to afford a child's medications because of failure of the other parent to make child support payments. Medical–legal partnerships address these types of situations in working toward the ultimate goal of increasing a patient's ability to manage disease, he explained.

Another example of wraparound services is the inclusion of mental health, child care, family services, and vocational training in substance use disorder treatment clinics. Menachemi and colleagues published a study of FQHCs in inner-city Indianapolis, Indiana, where wraparound services included social work, dietician assistance, and patient navigation (Vest et al., 2018). These wraparound services reduced hospitalizations and emergency department visits in the years following the rollout of these services. Another study that focused on nutritionists found that seeing a dietician can improve a patient's diet quality, diabetes outcomes, and weight loss (Mitchell et al., 2017). The co-location of behavioral health wraparound services in primary care settings was the focus of another study, which found that this co-location can reduce wait times for treatments and increase both patient engagement in care and patient use of needed services (Possemato et al., 2018).

Challenges to Adoption of Wraparound Services

Both rural and urban areas are seeing a low uptake of wraparound services, noted Menachemi. He attributed this to the historic fee-for-service incentive structure—a somewhat perverse incentive structure that was implemented because most providers and facilities are set up to address acute issues rather than the chronic conditions that are largely driven by the SDOH. This effectively disincentivized wraparound services, despite the fact that wraparound services can reduce the need for future services that are costlier. The study conducted by Menachemi and colleagues on wraparound services in an Indianapolis FQHC indicated an average annual cost savings of approximately $2 million (Vest et al., 2018). He noted that under a fee-for-service structure, cost savings are actually a reduction in revenue, whereas under full capitation,[14] they represent true savings for the provider. Therefore, the financial incentives

---

[14] Under capitation, "providers receive a fixed per person (or 'capitated') payment that covers all health care services over a defined time period, adjusted for each patient's expected needs, and are also held accountable for high-quality outcomes." See James and Poulsen (2016).

and reimbursement model used will affect whether or not the use of wraparound services is incentivized. He said that wraparound services are most frequently geared toward vulnerable groups, as this model is more readily adopted by FQHCs and clinics that disproportionately cater to vulnerable individuals. The focus of these settings, reflected in their goals and mission, is usually on ameliorating challenges and not necessarily on generating revenue.

Implications of Wraparound Services for Rural Health

Menachemi suggested that in many ways, rural settings may be ideal for wraparound services because rural populations tend to have many needs stemming from unfavorable social determinants. Therefore, he suggested exploring ways to integrate the expertise of various providers working to mitigate the unfavorable ramifications of SDOH. He described several studies that illustrate the potential benefit of implementing wraparound services in rural areas. One study looked at a dental clinic that used the wraparound service of transportation assistance, finding that dental treatment completion rates increased with transportation assistance in place (Larson et al., 2019). The study also found that most wraparound services are supported via grants or philanthropy, making them vulnerable to funding disruptions. Menachemi said that this type of vulnerability is more likely when the financial model of delivering care is not aligned with the engagement of wraparound services. Another study looked at substance use disorder treatment centers in both rural and urban areas (Bond Edmond et al., 2015). Centers in rural locations were far less likely to offer wraparound services than their urban counterparts because of challenges in rural areas, including the stigma on behavioral health care issues (Pullmann et al., 2010). He said that many of the barriers to wraparound services in rural areas are the same barriers seen in accessing medical and primary care: transportation issues, limited funding, service availability, a shortage of wraparound service providers, and long distances between facilities all pose challenges to accessing wraparound services in rural locations.

Menachemi remarked that the issues that have historically impeded access to primary care and dental services are being overcome, which may provide an opportunity for wraparound services to play a role in enhancing care in rural areas. He added that telehealth—which is rapidly expanding due to the COVID-19 pandemic—could potentially be used as a platform for delivering wraparound services. The use of wraparound services via telemedicine has not yet been studied, but he suggested that it could be useful if geographic access is a limiting factor. However, telehealth may not be as helpful in relieving the financial barriers to service provision in many rural communities, so the proliferation of telehealth could widen disparities in rural areas if financial and other barriers prevent access (June-Ho Kim and Cole, 2020).

THE ROLE OF COMMUNITY HEALTH WORKERS IN ADDRESSING THE NEEDS OF RURAL AMERICANS

Timothy Callaghan from the Southwest Rural Health Research Center at Texas A&M University focused his presentation on the role of the CHW in addressing the needs of rural Americans and the unique barriers they face in accessing health services. He presented data to define CHW roles, explored differences between CHWs in urban and rural environments, highlighted challenges in the growing CHW field, and described CHW efforts to combat the COVID-19 pandemic.

Overview of Community Health Workers

CHWs are individuals who help bridge the gap between the public—including the most vulnerable members of the community—and the health and social services that are available, Callaghan explained. CHWs are distinct from many other health care providers in that CHWs often come from the communities in which they serve. Being a community member enables CHWs to promote trust within the community and connect vulnerable individuals to the services they need. He noted that the literature on CHWs as well as anecdotal personal experiences demonstrate that CHWs often possess unique cultural competence and a personal understanding of their communities and their patients, which equips CHWs to help those patients overcome barriers to accessing health care services. The CHW workforce is growing rapidly, he added. The Bureau of Labor Statistics projected that the CHW workforce would increase by up to 13 percent between 2018 and 2028.[15] In Texas, the number of CHWs in the field has increased by more than 500 percent in just the past few years (Callaghan et al., 2019).

Community Health Worker Roles

To describe the roles of CHWs in rural and urban settings in the United States, Callaghan used two sources of original data from research

---

[15] More information about the CHW job outlook is available at https://www.bls.gov/OOH/community-and-social-service/health-educators.htm#tab-6 (accessed July 31, 2020).

conducted with support from the Federal Office of Rural Health Policy.[16] The first source is a series of focus groups held with CHWs in rural and urban parts of California, Florida, Massachusetts, and Minnesota in 2018 and 2019. The second came from a large 2019 survey of more than 1,400 CHW participants from 45 states, Puerto Rico, and the District of Columbia. Callaghan explained that when CHWs were asked to describe their own roles during the focus groups and surveys, three themes emerged: (1) linking clients to resources, (2) focusing on SDOH, and (3) providing insights to other health care providers about clients that might otherwise be missed (see Box 4-1). CHWs in both urban and rural areas highlighted their roles in linking clients to resources, suggesting that in being a part of the communities they serve, CHWs are enabled to better understand the needs of clients because they may have experienced these needs themselves. The CHW role of serving as a bridge to agencies and services is similar in both rural and urban areas. He added that the resources that CHWs help their clients link up with often extend beyond health care resources. This is evident in another role that survey respondents and focus group participants described: addressing SDOH. Rather than focusing on one single area, CHWs fill in a variety of gaps, from addressing SDOH to navigating aspects of the health care system to providing links to wraparound services. The third role that emerged from the focus groups is that CHWs can provide insights about patients that might be missed by other health care providers. Not only do CHWs understand the communities they serve, they also enter the homes of patients, which provides the opportunity to glean critical holistic information about their patients' lives that may be affecting their health.

Community Health Workers in Rural Versus Urban Settings

The increasing numbers of CHWs are filling a vital role in the health care system, said Callaghan. The value of CHWs extends to rural areas, where they can help patients address the considerable barriers rural Americans face in accessing health care services. These barriers include transportation issues, limited numbers of providers, barriers to hospital access, and limited social programs. Callaghan suggested that if CHWs are uniquely positioned to help link clients to resources, they might be even more important in rural areas where those resources are scarce. The

---

[16] These were original data sets collected for a Federal Office of Rural Health Policy–funded project. The project description can be found at https://www.ruralhealthresearch.org/projects/100002452 (accessed April 9, 2021), and the first policy brief about this can be found at https://srhrc.tamhsc.edu/docs/chw-policy-brief.pdf (accessed April 9, 2021).

> **BOX 4-1**
> **Community Health Workers' Reflections on Their Roles**
>
> *On linking clients with resources:*
>
> "We are this bridge between the agencies, their resources, and the community. *Promotores* [CHWs] are very successful ... because we have this connection with people, we go to their level, we understand people because we belong to the community, we know their needs, a lot of times we experience them." (Community health worker in rural California)
>
> "I would say ... linking clients to resources. That would be to providers whether it's medical, dental, where you can get vision, where you can get a hearing screening, diapers, whatever the resources that the clients need. Linking them to those resources." (Community health worker in Los Angeles, California)
>
> *On addressing social determinants of health:*
>
> "We help with insurance, and then we help with homelessness, and then we help with food, and then we help with moving, and then we help with dental access, and behavioral health access. And that's all before noon." (Community health worker in Minnesota)
>
> "If you're worried about homelessness, if you're worried about where your next meal's coming from, or child care, or all these things that are directly related to your family, you're not focusing on your health. You're focusing on these things. So, that's where we come into play.... Nine times out of ten, they don't even identify anything health related. It's mostly social." (Community health worker in Boston, Massachusetts)
>
> *On providing insight about clients that might otherwise be missed:*
>
> "Especially if you go into the home, you had the opportunity to see the whole client, not just the COPD [chronic obstructive pulmonary disease], not just the diabetes, not just the person who is vulnerable.... You had the opportunity to see the person as they live. And that's something that your doctor doesn't get to see or your nurse in the hospital doesn't get to see. You just have a better understanding of where they are." (Community health worker in rural Florida)
>
> "Then we can go back and relay to the doctor and the nurses what kind of problems [patients have].... They [medical providers] actually get an insight on who their patients are and get to know them a little bit better because of us." (Community health worker in Massachusetts)
>
> SOURCE: Callaghan presentation, June 24, 2020.

CHW survey data indicate that 28.9 percent of CHWs primarily serve rural clients, while 43.4 percent primarily work with urban clients.

Callaghan reported that in both rural and urban areas, CHWs are employed in a variety of settings: hospitals, doctors' offices, clinics, nonprofits, academic institutions, and community outreach organizations. However, certain trends emerge when looking at the percentages of urban and rural CHWs working in each of these settings. For example, urban CHWs are more likely to work in hospitals and in community outreach settings than their rural counterparts. He attributed this to a lack of hospitals in rural areas and the long distances rural CHWs would have to travel to go door to door for community outreach. Instead, rural CHWs are more likely to be working in doctors' offices and clinics. Additionally, they are more likely than urban CHWs to work in roles that are harder to define or categorized as "other" because their work does not fit neatly into the specified category descriptions.

The demographic characteristics of rural and urban CHWs also differ, said Callaghan. The average age of rural CHWs is about 3 years older than their urban counterparts, which is consistent with the demographics of the general population living in rural areas. Rural CHWs also tend to have lower levels of education, with 42.3 percent holding a bachelor's degree compared to 52.3 percent of urban CHWs. An overwhelming majority (90 percent) of CHWs in the survey data were female. This trend is even more pronounced in rural areas, where only 6.2 percent of CHWs are male, than in urban areas, where 12.5 percent are male.

Beyond demographics, the work performed by CHWs looks different in urban versus rural areas. Callaghan highlighted two key differences that were evident in the focus groups. The first is that urban CHWs tend to be specialists that are highly focused on a specific task (e.g., enrolling individuals in a program), a certain subpopulation, or a specific disease like diabetes. In contrast, rural CHWs tend to be generalists. They are more likely to address all of the needs of the individuals because there may be no equivalent health care workers in the area to address patients' various needs. As a CHW in rural Minnesota remarked:

> In an urban setting often they're adding a CHW specialized in diabetes, specialized in prenatal care, specialized in something that they can really train that individual, and they have a large enough population that they can serve just that population, and that it really makes that difference in those urban areas. And I think the big thing I've seen different for us in a rural area is we have to be very generalist.

Callaghan noted that in addition to the reduced number of programs in rural areas, CHWs in these regions also have fewer resources available to which their clients can be linked. Even where there are programs available in rural areas, they tend to be more limited than in cities. In contrast, patients in some urban areas can be overwhelmed with the number of resources that are potentially available to them, as was articulated by an urban CHW:

> Everybody in Boston that has something going on has been offered some kind of program. Really, they're so overwhelmed by, "Oh, we have five different programs, I don't want another program."

In the same state of Massachusetts, a rural CHW responded:

> In rural areas here, there's less transportation, there's less resources, there's less funding. Sometimes it can be trying. We have a program right now that CHWs work with: if you're struggling with food, we can give you a gift card for a certain amount, each person in the house, but that's limited. We can't give it to everybody, and everybody at some point has problems with food insecurities.

Challenges in Building the Workforce of Community Health Workers

Callaghan explained that beyond the lack of resources available for rural clients, there are challenges within the way CHW jobs are structured. Even as this field grows, CHW study participants repeatedly noted key barriers to expanding the workforce in ways that would particularly benefit rural America. Two of the barriers emerged as most prominent in the study. The first issue is the variety of terminology used to describe CHW positions. Callaghan and his team identified dozens of terms for CHWs such as *promotor(a)*, health educator, and health navigator. The absence of a widely accepted nomenclature poses challenges to the professionalization of this field, as terminology is important in the creation of regulations and consistent standards. Without an agreed-upon term for CHWs, confusion might arise as to whether state and federal laws and regulations are applicable. For example, if a law is passed in Texas focused on CHWs, people working under the title of *promotor(a)* or health educator may be unclear as to whether the law applies to them.

The second major challenge repeatedly cited by CHWs was payment, with respect to both sources of funding and practices for billing. Many CHWs reported working in grant-funded positions that do not provide them with long-term security, because their jobs may disappear with the end of the grant cycle. Challenges in billing practices relate to the lack of billing codes for services to address SDOH and other social factors of health outcomes, said Callaghan. The challenges involved in funding CHW positions can discourage health care providers from hiring CHWs despite the improvements they can have on patient outcomes.

Community Health Worker Efforts to Combat COVID-19

Callaghan noted that extensive efforts to train CHWs across the country to address the global pandemic began almost as soon as COVID-19 started spreading across the United States. In Texas, for example, the first training sessions were held in early March, including a session in South Texas for *promotores* along the Texas–Mexico border. The National Association of Community Health Workers,[17] the American Public Health Association's CHW Section,[18] and various training centers across the country have been promoting CHW workshops to help them fight the coronavirus pandemic and to ensure that CHWs are staying safe.

Callaghan stated that research by his team suggests that CHWs are taking on new roles in response to the pandemic. A prominent role is contract tracing, which is vital to understanding the spread of the disease. Callaghan said that CHWs are well qualified for this role because they come from the communities they serve, enabling them to provide culturally appropriate support and establish trust with patients in a way that might be more difficult for contract tracers from outside the community. CHWs' pandemic-expanded roles also include tasks such as making masks for vulnerable individuals and picking up groceries for individuals who might be too vulnerable to go into stores themselves. As CHWs continue to perform their previous roles, they have had to adapt their work in order to practice social distancing—including increased use of teleconferencing technologies to safely connect to clients.

Certain challenges that have emerged during the pandemic particularly affect rural CHWs, said Callaghan. Because of a lack of Internet access in many rural areas, some rural CHWs cannot use teleconferencing with their clients, making it more difficult to provide socially distanced services. In addition, many CHWs have been laid off because of the reduced funding many organizations have experienced during the pandemic. Additionally, billing for in-person services addressing SDOH is even more difficult when these services are provided online.

---

[17] More information about the National Association of Community Health Workers is available at https://nachw.org (accessed August 6, 2020).

[18] More information about the American Public Health Association's CHW Section is available at https://www.apha.org/apha-communities/member-sections/community-health-workers (accessed August 6, 2020).

DISCUSSION

Telehealth Mental Health Services During the Pandemic

Morris asked about the role of telehealth services in response to the COVID-19 pandemic—particularly the delivery of mental health services for youth and older adults. Calac replied that at the Indian Health Council facility where he works, the behavioral health wing continues to serve clients at nearly the same capacity (roughly 90 percent) of pre-pandemic levels through the use of telehealth services for both adult and pediatric client populations. He noted that a disadvantage of delivering mental health services through telehealth, especially for pediatric patients, is that it limits the amount of observation data that a clinician can collect. However, telehealth sessions have the benefit of allowing the clinician to observe pediatric clients in their home environments, which is helpful for behavioral health services. The patient response to the shift to telehealth has been varied, added Calac. Some individuals are frustrated by the platforms and by the limited capacity in some areas. Creative efforts have been made to address these issues by using nonsecure platforms that patients may be more familiar with (e.g., FaceTime, Zoom) in between scheduled sessions. Other clients enjoy being in their home environment for telehealth appointments because the setting feels less formal, he noted.

Rural Health Care Financing Challenges

Morris asked about the types of research that may be needed to determine which hospitals are at the highest risk of closure, about the role of the COVID-19 pandemic in determining that risk, and about long-term improvements that are needed beyond basic reimbursement changes and pilot programs. Moore responded that financially fragile systems are vulnerable because they lack reserves, so any disruption can heavily impact vulnerable entities. The stressors that came with the pandemic, like canceled outpatient procedures, had an immediate negative effect on the finances of rural facilities. He explained that these types of facilities generally are not structured to provide a high volume of inpatient services, so their budgets are often based on outpatient procedures that may constitute 60 to 80 percent of their total business.

At the same time that rural facilities were seeing a decline in patients, urban areas were working to handle surges in patients with COVID-19, noted Moore. Consequently, underutilized rural hospitals were identified in some discussions as a potential resource to meet the increased need for medical care. Although these rural hospitals may be underutilized for elective and preplanned procedures, the surge capacity in rural hospitals might quickly disappear as individuals requiring hospital care for

COVID-19 in rural areas would still require the nearest ER. Moore was also concerned about the possible underreporting of COVID-19 cases in rural areas and the potential for rural health systems to exceed their capacity if rural regions experience the type of escalations in case numbers that were initially seen in urban centers. Moore added that long-standing disparities have become more prominent as the COVID-19 pandemic has begun to put additional stress on systems. Rural facilities already tend to have limited resources, and because smaller health facilities are often at the tail end of the supply chain, it is unclear whether health facilities will have the capacity to respond to a surge of COVID-19 cases in rural areas.

Calac remarked that the COVID-19 outbreak in the Navajo Nation in Arizona highlights the need for better processes around emergency preparedness in the future. He added that the pandemic affects different tribes in different ways, so improved processes and preparedness will need to be tailored to their specific settings. For instance, California has a general population of 33 million people and is home to more than 60 tribal entities, so an effective outbreak response in that state will look different than the response in Arizona. Regions in close proximity to the U.S.–Mexico border also face setting-specific challenges related to the COVID-19 pandemic. For instance, it has been difficult to translate and implement social distancing policies in border towns in Texas, where hospitals have seen an influx of patients from across the U.S.–Mexico border. Similarly, southern San Diego County has a much higher COVID-19 infection rate than northern San Diego County, suggesting that proximity to the border may exacerbate certain challenges faced by communities affected by COVID-19.

Menachemi contended that 70–80 percent of all of the challenges in the U.S. health care system stem from chronic underfunding and chronic underappreciation for public health, which put a strain on vulnerable facilities. He suggested that the COVID-19 pandemic may present a critical opportunity to rethink decades-old challenges in public health—even if it means political fallout for some leaders—and to implement holistic changes to the health care system at large.

Morris remarked that issues of structural urbanism, rural hospitals, hospital closures, and pick-your-provider services all relate to the central issue of health financing. Small tweaks in financing or health systems, such as increasing reimbursement by a small percentage, will not adequately address the situation. Menachemi agreed and responded that tweaking reimbursement within current structures would not be sufficient, as "reimbursement" implies medical care reimbursement rather than health care reimbursement. He added that the United States does a much better job at providing medical services than keeping people healthy or preventing diagnosed diseases from becoming more severe.

He suggested that the concept of health should be infused into the way society perceives health care, because many people think of health care merely as better medical care, but an insurance card does not solve life problems that are exacerbating one's health issues; it only helps patients cope better with the health issues they have, and it is not the most cost-effective method of promoting health, he added.

Callaghan said the current paradigm of the health care system is focused on profit maximization, which will continue to lead to more problems in rural areas. When profit maximization is the goal, rural areas are at a disadvantage because health care work in rural areas is typically less profitable than operating large urban hospitals. Callaghan suggested incentive structures need to be changed so that both health needs and the SDOH are addressed. He predicted that given current conditions and the trends of hospital closures, the health of rural communities will likely worsen owing to factors such as the need to travel longer distances for care.

Coordinating Care in Rural Areas

Morris questioned whether better use of wraparound services and CHWs could help ensure that care is coordinated, especially after people traveling long distances for specialty care return to their rural communities. Although his presentation focused on licensed or credentialed individuals, Menachemi clarified that CHWs certainly fit the definition of wraparound service providers. With the shortage of traditional wraparound service providers in rural areas, CHWs who are already working as generalists could feasibly be quickly trained to do the jobs that a half dozen professionals would perform in settings with more resources. However, he cautioned that this is a "path of least resistance" in that rather than building a health care workforce of highly trained individuals in rural areas, CHWs with less training become even more overburdened. This could perpetuate the problems of structural urbanism, he added.

Callaghan noted a debate in the CHW community over training and education. Many CHWs say they do not want additional training and education, because they value being a part of the community and feel that training would shift them from being a community member to being an "other." This gives rise to the question of whether additional training and education would affect the way patients relate to CHWs. He added that the effective provision of wraparound services in rural communities—for rural patients who have transferred home from large urban hospitals, for example—requires the type of robust coordination of care and communication between urban and rural health providers that is not commonplace.

Leveraging the Strengths of Rural Areas and Tribal Nations

Morris asked about the strengths of tribal nations and rural areas that policy makers should better understand. Moore responded that "rural areas are resource restricted, but they're relationship rich." He suggested that a strong sense of community and responsibility are rural strengths that would contribute to the delivery of effective care if needed changes could be made to the health care system. He used the analogy of electrical infrastructure to point out that governments take responsibility for running electrical lines in rural areas, but property owners are often responsible for the last quarter mile connecting their properties to the public infrastructure. Similarly, social services are needed in rural communities to manage health before expensive medical issues arise. Rural communities can rise to meet this challenge if there is proper health infrastructure in place, he suggested. A market where efficiency is driven by volume will not work in rural areas, Moore said. Rural communities do not have more volume to contribute to the system, so efficiency has to be driven by decreasing use of services in situations where it can be avoided. He suggested that CHWs and social services can contribute in this regard by addressing issues early on and preventing them from developing into expensive medical issues. Moore said the relationship-rich culture of rural communities is well equipped to carry out this type of early intervention.

Calac agreed that strong social structures, as well as the component of resiliency, have persisted in rural communities. This has allowed people to rely on one another for support in facing challenges related to accessing health care, he said. Unfortunately, this strength has proven to be an Achilles heel in the face of the pandemic, as individuals accustomed to relying on one another are being asked to stay at home and risk compounding their geographic isolation with social isolation. However, he suggested that the ability to tap into their resiliency will allow rural people to persevere. CHWs and wraparound services are another strength, he added. Physicians may only be able to see an individual for 15 minutes at a time, but sending a public health worker, a public health nurse, or a dietician to work with a client in person or via telehealth allows for the provision of a higher level of care to the community.

Morris asked why so little research has been conducted on the benefits to rural population health of coordinated care that includes wraparound services and CHWs. Menachemi responded that in most other developed nations, social workers do not deal with health care issues, but in the United States, social workers are patching up gaps in the health care system. He suggested that this is one of the many problems caused by the chronic underappreciation and underfunding of public health. In contrast to countries with well-organized and well-functioning health care systems that treat medicine and public health as two sides of the same coin, in the United States they are treated as different structures that require different training. Most people in the medical care delivery system do not interact with their local public health agency and have little interaction with their state agency, with the exception of data reporting required by law. Menachemi suggested that there is much room for partnerships and innovation in rural areas. By leveraging the strengths of relationships and trust in rural communities, innovations could be developed in rural areas and then scaled up to urban settings, he added.

Morris asked about data sources to better understand and scale up social services support structures. Menachemi suggested that the fields of implementation science and health services research could contribute, but the "elephant in the room" is that social services are being funded unsustainably through charity, philanthropy, and grants instead of being built into the bedrock of the health care systems in rural communities.

5

Assessment and Implementation Strategies for Improving the Health of Rural Populations

The fourth session of the workshop focused on the assessment and implementation of strategies for improving the health of rural populations, including the community health needs assessment (CHNA) tool, the Minnesota Integrating Behavioral Health project, rural development hubs, and strategies to catalyze innovation in sustainability and financing of rural population health. The session was moderated by Allen Smart from PhilanthropywoRx.

COMMUNITY HEALTH NEEDS ASSESSMENT

Darrold Bertsch from Sakakawea Medical Center (SMC) and Coal Country Community Health Center (CCCHC) discussed how the CHNA tool can be used to support population health efforts. He described the CHNA process and how it has been applied to inform organizational planning and collaborative assessment activities. CHNA is a tool that health care entities use to define their service area, identify the specific needs in that area, and facilitate planning to meet the health care needs within that area. Through a systematic process that draws on community input and support, the CHNA tool can identify health needs and health systems issues through data and information gathering and analysis. Bertsch added that CHNAs are conducted to identify and prioritize health needs within a community, which can provide justification for the allocation of resources based on the needs that are identified during the assessment process.

CHNAs are routinely conducted by a variety of entities and organizations, said Bertsch. For example, critical access hospitals (CAHs) must conduct CHNAs every 3 years, as mandated by the Patient Protection and Affordable Care Act, in order to identify community needs and move toward addressing them. Public health entities are required to conduct CHNAs for accreditation purposes and, more importantly, to inform the development of community health improvement plans that enable public health units to address community-specific needs. The Health Resources and Services Administration (HRSA) requires community health centers to use CHNAs—both for grant applications and for subsequent reporting from grant applications—to identify community needs and how those needs are being met in the scope of services provided by that health center. Bertsch noted that CHNAs are sometimes conducted independently without necessarily linking together to identify needs and work collaboratively to address them. However, the communities and organizations that tend to be most successful in using CHNAs are those where the needs assessments are conducted collaboratively and followed by collaborative planning.

Community Health Needs Assessment Process

Bertsch provided an overview of the CHNA process (see Box 5-1).[1] The process begins with reflecting and strategizing about the overarching goals to be accomplished through the needs assessment. The next step is to identify and engage with a variety of stakeholders who will be providing input and participating in the CHNA process (e.g., health care providers, local clergy, government agencies). Then, the community is defined based on the service area of the organization or multiple organizations participating in the assessment. Next, data are collected to identify needs using various types of strategies, including individual surveys, individual interviews, focus groups, or information available online, such as county health rankings. The data are then analyzed to prioritize community health issues through a series of meetings with smaller groups, followed by larger group meetings. The results of the entire scope of the assessment are then documented and communicated to stakeholders. This process yields a package of documents that serves as the guide for the remainder of the CHNA cycle; the success of the CHNA process is dependent on stakeholders making use of these documents. Next, the implementation phase begins. Using the results from the CHNA, stakeholders develop and begin to execute implementation strategies. The final

---

[1] More information about the community health needs assessment process is available at https://www.healthycommunities.org/resources/community-health-assessment-toolkit (accessed September 8, 2020).

> **BOX 5-1**
> **Community Health Needs Assessment Process**
>
> Step 1: Reflect and strategize.
> Step 2: Identify and engage stakeholders.
> Step 3: Define the community.
> Step 4: Collect and analyze data.
> Step 5: Prioritize community health issues.
> Step 6: Document and communicate results.
> Step 7: Plan implementation strategies.
> Step 8: Implement strategies.
> Step 9: Evaluate progress.
>
> SOURCES: Bertsch presentation, June 25, 2020; https://www.healthycommunities.org/resources/community-health-assessment-toolkit (accessed September 8, 2020).

phase is ongoing monitoring and evaluating of progress toward the goals that have been identified through the CHNA process. Bertsch added that if health priorities change as strategies are being implemented, implementation strategies need to be adjusted accordingly to meet the community's current health care needs.

Use of Community Health Needs Assessment Findings for Strategic Planning

Bertsch described how CHNA findings can be used for strategic planning and implementation. CHNA findings are used for strategic planning both for individual organizations and for collective planning within service areas. It tends to be more effective when health care entities in a community work collectively to develop strategic plans and then hold each other accountable to facilitate, implement, and monitor the initiatives developed during the strategic planning process. CHNA findings can also be used to collaborate with local public health units to develop and implement community health improvement plans. Through subsequent monitoring and regular meetings to review progress, local population health committees can use the CHNA findings to adjust strategic plans as needed. Bertsch emphasized that coordinated and collaborative assessment and planning are critical for ensuring that the CHNA process produces the greatest possible community benefit. He added that in some states, CHNA results are aggregated for use in statewide planning efforts. For instance, the Center for Rural Health in North Dakota aggregates CHNA data from individual providers to provide statewide data on health needs. This allows stakeholders to compare their communities' health needs and priorities with state averages and with the needs and priorities of other communities.

Application of Community Health Needs Assessment in North Dakota

Bertsch described the practical application of a collaborative CHNA and planning process that was conducted in North Dakota, and he explained how that process benefited SMC in Hazen, North Dakota, and CCCHC in Beulah, North Dakota. SMC and CCCHC are both 501(c)(3) not-for-profit corporations that serve a 4,000-square-mile rural service area in West Central North Dakota with a population of 15,000. Energy is the major industry in this service area. CCCHC was designated as a federally qualified health center in 2003; it comprises four service delivery sites and offers medical, behavioral health, and visiting nurse services. SMC is a 13-bed critical access hospital that offers hospital, hospice, palliative care, and basic care services.

The SMC and CCCHC collaborative CHNA and planning process began in 2011, said Bertsch. The process benefited from integrated leadership and governance for the two facilities, which ensured that both the health center and the hospital remain aligned in terms of vision and strategic initiatives. Multiple community partners were involved in the initial needs assessment. In addition to core partners including SMC, CCCHC, the public health unit, a skilled nursing facility, and emergency medical services providers, additional participants included state and local governments, businesses and industry representatives, school administrations, and other community representatives.

Bertsch outlined several benefits of the collaborative CHNA and planning process in North Dakota. The process benefited from both individual and collective efforts to identify community needs and move forward with developing and implementing the strategic planning process through a collaborative and coordinated community health improvement plan. The population health committee plays a valuable role in monitoring progress and adjusting the implementation plan based on changes in the service area's health needs, which benefits from a collaborative process that aligns efforts across partner entities. Bertsch remarked that the CHNA process was instrumental in creating a "patient-centered medical neighborhood of care" among organizations involved in the process. This has improved financial performance, clinical outcomes, and quality metrics, and it has enhanced collaborative care, care coordination, and transitions of care. Care coordinators at each organization are able to work together across initiatives because the organizations are collectively involved in the needs identification and planning processes. This collaborative process has also established a foundation for additional initiatives, Bertsch noted. For instance, SMC and CCCHC have jointly implemented a new electronic medical record system.

Partner organizations in the service area are also participating in value-based care for Medicare and commercial models. This has provided a framework for a patient–family advisory council that includes representatives from each entity in the service area, as well as a group of patients who have used hospital, clinic, long-term care, and emergency medical services. Such initiatives would not have been possible without the collaborative approach to the CHNA process from the outset, he noted, and such an approach will likely serve the community well in addressing future needs. Bertsch added that the framework for collaborative planning and collaboration established by the CHNA process has been helpful in addressing local needs and facilitating responsiveness during the coronavirus disease 2019 (COVID-19) pandemic.

MINNESOTA INTEGRATED BEHAVIORAL HEALTH PROGRAM TO SUPPORT POPULATION HEALTH

Rhonda Barcus from the National Rural Health Resource Center[2] discussed the development of the Minnesota Integrated Behavioral Health (IBH) program to support population health. The Minnesota IBH program was funded by the Minnesota Department of Health's Office of Rural Health and Primary Care as part of a Minnesota Flex Program grant focused on population health. The Department of Health analyzed 59 CHNA findings from Minnesota communities and found that one of the most frequently cited needs was for behavioral health. Specifically, these CHNAs demonstrated a statewide need to build community partnerships and integrate behavioral health and outreach. This was consistent with aggregated local public health department findings, which identified access to behavioral health services as the greatest need statewide. Thus, the Department of Health decided to systematically coordinate behavioral health with general care, said Barcus, because integrating mental health, substance abuse, and primary care services produces the best outcomes and has been shown to be the most effective approach to caring for people with multiple health care needs.

---

[2] The National Rural Health Resource Center is a nonprofit organization dedicated to sustaining and improving health care in rural communities. As the nation's leading technical assistance and knowledge center in rural health, the center focuses on five core areas: transition to value and population health, collaboration and partnership, performance improvement, health information technology, and workforce.

The program was developed in collaboration with the hospitals that would be participating in the program, which were focused on tightening and improving care coordination practices for people in the community with behavioral health issues. From the hospital's perspective, the intention was to provide sufficiently high-quality supportive care to individuals with behavioral health issues that they are less likely to experience a crisis requiring them to seek care in a hospital's emergency department (ED). Although many communities were already offering a range of behavioral health services, those services were often siloed with minimal collaboration among providers. Barcus added that the development of the IBH brought together a range of different organizations focused on behavioral health and mitigating the potentially negative effects of social determinants of health (SDOH)—including competing organizations, in some cases—to determine how to best serve the people in the community.

Minnesota Integrated Behavioral Health Program Tool Kit

One of the results of the collaborative IBH project was the development of the IBH tool kit.[3] Barcus explained that the tool kit was designed both to provide detailed information for entities seeking to address behavioral health in their communities and to serve as a generic process for addressing other population health issues, such as diabetes or heart disease. The tool kit provides details about the IBH project process, including information about the readiness assessment, selection process, technical assistance, evaluation of project outcomes, and lessons learned. The IBH project worked with three cohorts of hospitals across the state—rolling out one cohort each year.

Technical Assistance to Hospital Cohorts

Barcus described the technical assistance provided to participating hospitals throughout the IBH process, which is detailed in the tool kit. For each cohort, a kickoff workshop brought together representatives of the participating hospitals. Next, each hospital in the cohort received an onsite visit to conduct community strategic planning. Quarterly peer calls allowed all of the hospitals in the cohort to share accomplishments, identify barriers and challenges, and brainstorm collaboratively about ways to address those issues. Hospitals also benefited from the provision

---

[3] The IBH project ran from 2015 to 2019, with cohort 1 in 2015, cohort 2 in 2016, cohort 3 in 2017, and a stigma project in 2018. More information about the IBH tool kit is available at https://www.ruralcenter.org/rhi/mn-ibh (accessed July 21, 2020).

of technical assistance as needed, as well as from educational webinars and workshops focused on sustainability and support for data collection.

Evaluation of Project Outcomes

Barcus described how the IBH project evaluated outcomes. The project used an outcome evaluation process developed by the National Rural Health Resource Center called recommendation adoption progress (RAP) reports. This process seeks to "tell the whole story" by including measurable outcomes as well as other concerns. As part of this process, the hospitals conduct regular interviews with project leaders throughout implementation and demonstrate ways in which the project has become embedded in their hospital culture. The IBH project teams conducted interviews with hospital teams to gain a holistic picture of how projects were being implemented and embedded in the hospital's culture. To help keep teams focused and motivated, RAP interviews are held quarterly. This holistic picture can be used to inform future projects in other hospitals, noted Barcus. Additionally, this evaluation process can be used to help maintain hospitals' momentum and promote accountability in realizing progress. For instance, if a hospital has not made the planned progress between quarterly evaluation calls, then the call can be used to help the hospital establish steps to achieve their goals.

Barcus explained that hospitals participating in the IBH project were also asked to develop their own measures—based on the specific populations that each hospital serves—in four general categories: (1) hospital-specific use of services measure, (2) hospital-specific cost-of-services measure, (3) hospital-specific health outcomes measure, and (4) hospital-specific individual measure. For example, a hospital-specific use of services measure might be specified as a measure of how many people with a certain type of behavioral health diagnosis are reporting to the hospital's ED each quarter. That hospital might then choose a cost-of-services measure that tracks the cost of services for each individual with that diagnosis who reported to the ED that quarter. These hospital-specific measures are discussed during quarterly evaluation calls. Barcus presented a practical example from one of the participating hospitals, which created a roving therapist position after finding that inmates in the local jail with depression and anxiety were presenting at the ED for treatment during crisis. The roving therapist began visiting the jail to counsel inmates with depression and anxiety to help prevent them from reaching a crisis point by providing them with longer-term supportive care. Over the subsequent year, the number of patients brought to the ED from the jail decreased and there were no inpatient psychiatric transfers among inmates in the jail who were seen by the roving therapist.

Integrating Behavioral Health: Measurable Outcomes and Promising Practices

Barcus outlined measurable outcomes used by hospitals that participated in the Minnesota IBH project to assess whether behavioral health was successfully integrated:[4]

- Increased access to behavioral health services,
- Increased discharge to home,[5]
- Decreased transfers to inpatient settings,
- Decreased cost of transferring ED patients as well as cost of ED visits,
- Decreased ED visits and admissions,
- Decreased mental health holds,
- Decreased Patient Health Questionnaire (PHQ-9) scores at 6-month follow-up, and
- Decreased jail psychiatric transfers.

Barcus also described examples of promising practices that participating hospitals identified as driving meaningful changes within hospitals. One of the most effective practices identified was stakeholder collaboration, which is the practice of identifying and engaging with stakeholders in the planning of projects. Resource directories were effective in allowing providers and consumers to identify available opportunities to access services. She noted that hospitals often began the IBH process presuming that more behavioral health resources were needed. However, establishing a resource directory can demonstrate that there are actually sufficient resources in place that consumers and providers are unaware of due to siloing and lack of collaboration. To help simplify the release process, some participating hospitals created a universal release of information that includes a list of potential agencies that will support a client's care release.[6] The use of community navigators can provide support and help ensure that clients are following their treatment plans and/or taking their medications. Another promising practice was the use of mobile crisis teams that report directly to clients' homes to assess and deescalate situations. For hospitals that rely on the police to transport patients to an

---

[4] More information about the Minnesota IBH project is available at https://www.ruralcenter.org/rhi/mn-ibh (accessed July 21, 2020).

[5] This outcome measures how often patients can be sent home instead of being discharged. Hospitals consider it a success when patients can be sent home instead of being discharged to inpatient care; these cases are referred to as "discharge to home."

[6] A sample universal release of information form can be found at https://www.ruralcenter.org/sites/default/files/Luverne%20Consent%20ROI.pdf (accessed July 21, 2020).

inpatient medical facility—often at great cost to the community—decommissioned police vehicles that have been purchased or donated can be used in lieu of an ambulance.

Barcus noted that implementing the Make It OK campaign is a promising practice for fighting stigma.[7] Across all three hospital cohorts in the IBH project, stigma around mental illness, behavioral health, and substance abuse was identified as one of the biggest barriers to good community care coordination. The Make It OK campaign has been used within and beyond hospitals to promote awareness and destigmatize mental illness and substance abuse.[8] In addition to using this campaign, other strategies for mitigating stigma include the formation of a committee of community partners to address stigma, engaging local institutions, and offering education and training on stigma reduction. Community collaboration is a key aspect of successful approaches to stigma reduction used by participating hospitals, Barcus added. In addition to strategies such as partnering with schools, churches, and businesses, some hospitals collaborated with music, art, and theater communities to create productions that would bring people together to help address the stigma of mental illness and substance abuse.

ROLE OF RURAL DEVELOPMENT HUBS AND POLICY IN CONNECTING RURAL DEVELOPMENT, HEALTH, AND OPPORTUNITY

Katharine Ferguson from The Aspen Institute Community Strategies Group discussed the role of rural development hubs and rural policy in connecting development, health, and opportunity in rural communities. She also suggested strategies to modernize federal rural policy and develop a stronger rural development ecosystem.

Influence of Community and Economic Development Efforts on Health

Ferguson highlighted the need to consider factors beyond clinical settings and health behaviors in advancing health, equity, and opportunity—this, in essence, is the thesis of population health. She noted that the underlying framework on which county-level health rankings and road

---

[7] See https://www.youtube.com/watch?v=KCL5YgNJTdw&feature=youtu.be (accessed September 21, 2021) and https://www.youtube.com/watch?v=2EiIwksKqQo&feature=youtu.be (accessed April 9, 2021).

[8] More information about the Make It OK campaign is available at https://makeitok.org (accessed July 21, 2020).

maps are based indicates that about 50 percent of health outcomes are related to social and economic factors (around 40 percent) and physical environment (about 10 percent),[9] and she emphasized the need to consider what it takes to create a healthy *place* where people feel they belong and can thrive, in addition to the more common focus on healthy *people* and individual opportunity.[10] Social and economic factors that span people and place include education, employment, income, family and social support, and community safety. Factors in the physical environment that are decidedly place focused include air and water quality as well as housing and transit.

Ferguson said that the concept of SDOH has been crucial in creating a structure and vocabulary for thinking beyond health care to health, well-being, and opportunity, but that the social determinants framework must continue to evolve to better reflect the full range of actors who are essential to creating an equitable, healthy, thriving, and sustainable place. Taking a broader lens means that actors, factors, and activities essential to health include community and economic development professionals, civic participation, tax and fiscal policy, structural racism, community building, place making and community planning decisions and the built environment, employers and workforce, and entrepreneurship and small business development in addition to the more commonly known actors and factors such as community health workers, schools and educators, day care providers, social service providers, safety and security providers, food assistance providers, and housing accessibility and affordability. In short, when a place—rather than a people—lens is applied to health, a wide range of systemic and structural factors ranging from racial justice to community planning and tax policy become essential to health.

Awareness is growing beyond public health and academic circles that *place*—where people live—is an important component of health and equity in the United States, with a critical intersection between race, class, and place. Some areas may have excellent schools, employers, transportation service, mental health services, and recreational opportunities, while others have subpar services or lack of services. Disparities have always existed, she noted, and the COVID-19 pandemic is making them more evident. The University of Michigan's Poverty Solutions Lab has developed a Multidimensional Index of Deep Disadvantage that measures

---

[9] More information about the County Health Rankings and Road Maps model is available at https://www.countyhealthrankings.org/explore-health-rankings/measures-data-sources/county-health-rankings-model?componentType=health-factor&componentId=25 (accessed July 22, 2020).

[10] Within this framework, about 30 percent of health outcomes are related to health behaviors (e.g., tobacco use, diet and exercise, alcohol and drug use, sexual activity) and 20 percent are related to clinical care, including access to care and quality of care.

five health status factors to assess what it is like to live in a particular place in the United States.[11] This index demonstrates that *place matters* and that great disparities exist across the country. For example, poverty is endemic and opportunity is limited in the Black Belt, in Appalachia, and in the *colonias* on the southwest U.S. border,[12] an area that is largely Indian country. Ferguson said that these areas should be evaluated with a broad lens in order to determine how structures and systems make it difficult to create healthy places and for individuals to realize opportunities in these regions:

> The cultural, historical, economic, and geographic context of place is essential and often points to regions where overcoming barriers to opportunity requires taking a much broader lens and think through how [to] look at the structures and the systems that are making it hard to realize opportunity.

Ferguson highlighted a set of rural and regional intermediary organizations that tend to be less visible as important developmental actors in communities and rural regions. These include community development financial institutions and credit unions created specifically to serve underserved regions, as well as community foundations, community colleges, community action agencies, regionally focused nonprofit organizations, value-chain coordinators, statewide rural organizations, social enterprise collaboratives and cooperatives, and regional councils of governments, among others. Ferguson noted that these organizations may not have an obvious place in the SDOH framework, but they are critical partners for making progress in population health by addressing root causes and effecting systemic change. A subset of those rural and regional intermediary organizations could be considered rural development hubs, she suggested.

Rural Development Hubs

Ferguson's organization, The Aspen Institute Community Strategies Group, has defined a rural development hub as "a place-rooted organization working hand in glove with people and organizations within

---

[11] More information about communities of deep disadvantage is available at https://poverty.umich.edu/projects/understanding-communities-of-deep-disadvantage (accessed July 22, 2020).

[12] The Texas Office of the Secretary of State defined the *colonias* as residential areas along the Texas–Mexico border that may lack basic living necessities like potable water, septic or sewer systems, electricity, paved roads, or safe and sanitary housing. More information about the *colonias* is available at https://mhpsalud.org/inside-texas-border-communities-colonias (accessed July 22, 2020).

and across a region to build inclusive wealth, increase local capacity, and create opportunities for better livelihoods, health, and well-being" in the report *Rural Development Hubs: Strengthening America's Rural Innovation Infrastructure* (The Aspen Institute Community Strategies Group, 2019). In developing the report, the group conducted interviews with leaders in 43 rural development hubs across the country that were representative in terms of geography, types of organization, and populations. The leaders were asked how they thought about their work, what challenges they face, and what would help them improve their work. Ferguson noted that a wide range of organizations can be considered rural development hubs, as already outlined. Although their work is critical for rural development, these intermediary organizations are not always easy to identify as potential partners in the current models used by public health organizations because they often work behind the scenes as partners to direct-service organizations and local organizations that public health is more likely to recognize.[13]

Outcome-Oriented, Wealth-Building Framework for Development

Rural development hubs may be radically different in terms of function and location, Ferguson said. However, a commonality among these organizations is their commitment to an asset-based approach to community and economic development rather than an overreliance on older approaches to economic development that often emphasize business recruitment and resource extraction. Instead, many rural development hubs are aligned with a wealth-building framework for development that is oriented around three outcomes:[14] (1) to grow multiple forms of capital, (2) to root ownership in the region, and (3) to improve livelihoods for those living on the margins. Specifically, these organizations tend to have a shared understanding of the need to recognize, invest in, and grow many kinds of capital—including individual, intellectual, social, natural, political, cultural, and financial capital—that are needed to create vibrant thriving communities and sustain economies. These organizations have a common interest in creating locally rooted wealth (not merely jobs), so that people in their regions will profit and experience better economic and health outcomes. Ferguson noted that locally rooted ownership creates more pathways for local-level ownership, control, and influence over economic drivers and for access to the wealth generated by those drivers. To improve the livelihoods of marginalized populations, these types of

---

[13] The Aspen Institute Community Strategies Group's report on rural development hubs includes tools that can be used to identify rural development hubs.

[14] For more information, see https://www.wealthworks.org (accessed October 28, 2020).

organizations aim to strengthen and improve livelihoods by providing high-quality, living-wage work and careers for all residents. They also focus on equity and inclusivity, aiming to improve the holistic livelihood of communities, added Ferguson.

Expanded Rural Hub Development Toolbox

Ferguson compared the toolbox for economic development, as traditionally construed, with the expanded toolbox that is common among rural development hubs. Traditional economic development tools include marketing a place or region, resource extraction (often timber, coal, or oil), and business recruitment through tax credits or investment-ready development (e.g., industrial parks). All of these tools may be used by rural development hubs, but their expanded toolbox also includes additional tools. These include systems thinking using a regional lens, a broader understanding of capital, community engagement with a focus on equity, and an emphasis on local ownership. More broadly, the expanded toolbox conceptualizes success in a way that focuses on health, resilience, high-quality jobs, and building and retaining local wealth.

Role of Rural Development Hubs in Addressing Social Determinants of Health

Ferguson emphasized that rural and regional intermediaries, such as rural development hubs, are essential partners in addressing structural barriers to progress and mitigating the negative consequences of SDOH in rural regions. They consider the whole system and engage a wide array of nontraditional partners among different sectors of the community to achieve positive outcomes in a way that is compatible with the population health. The unique lens and language of rural and regional intermediaries such as rural development hubs makes them an invaluable asset to those working on SDOH and population health. She quoted Patrick Woodie of the North Carolina Rural Center:

> Our aim is to create a place at the table for all parts of the community, especially those parts that may look different or have not always been included in the conversation. Inclusion cannot happen on its own. It must be an intentional part of any economic or community development strategy.

Developing a Stronger Rural Development Ecosystem

Ferguson emphasized that strategies are needed to encourage the development of more and stronger rural development hubs and engage them more broadly in development work. She described 10 routes to a stronger rural development ecosystem, which are organized into three forms of action: shifting mindsets, constructing or revising systems and policies, and building capacity (The Aspen Institute Community Strategies Group, 2019).

Shifting mindsets would benefit from (1) an understanding that addressing equity in the United States requires investments in rural America, (2) an increase in U.S. rural cultural competency, (3) trust in the know-how of rural development hubs, and (4) a reimagining of what *impact* means in rural contexts.

To construct or revise systems and policies, it would be useful to (5) detect and eradicate government systems and structures that disadvantage rural America, and (6) design policies and programs with rural implementation in mind.

To build capacity, it would be helpful to (7) support analysis and action at the regional level, (8) boost peer learning for hub staff and board leaders, (9) create pipelines and marketplaces that connect investors to America's rural development, and (10) structure investments and initiatives to strengthen and sustain system-changing organizations. In addition to these 10 routes for building a stronger rural development ecosystem, Ferguson called for the creation of a consensus vision and framework for rural community and economic development.

Strategies to Modernize Federal Rural Policy and Connect Health with Development

Ferguson explained that rural economies were hit hardest by the 2008 recession and have been the slowest to recover. In 2017, average rural employment was still 2 percent lower than it was in 2007.[15] Businesses were hit especially hard by the recession; in the first 4 years of recovery, counties with populations under 100,000 lost 17,500 businesses, while economies in counties with populations of 1 million or more gained 99,000 jobs (Ferguson et al., 2020). Existing racial, health, and economic disparities are being exacerbated by the COVID-19 pandemic, and it is critical that these health and economic issues be addressed concurrently. She suggested that events surrounding the COVID-19 pandemic support the claim that health and economic outcomes are integral and need to be addressed simultaneously.

A major challenge in supporting the economic development of rural

---

[15] More information about rural employment is available at https://www.ers.usda.gov/topics/rural-economy-population/employment-education/rural-employment-and-unemployment (accessed July 22, 2020).

communities is that federal rural policy is largely outdated, said Ferguson. While the pressures and opportunities faced by rural economies have radically changed, the existing federal architecture for rural policy is old—largely dating to the 1860s, 1930s, and 1960s—and designed for a different time (Ferguson et al., 2020). She suggested that population health advocates and other health advocates should join in advocating for the modernization of federal rural policy toward a rural policy framework that helps to achieve both economic and health goals. Ferguson presented five principles for reimagining federal policy in the COVID-19 era:

1. Support local ownership and strategies.
2. Invest in people and institutions.
3. Increase flexibility and align federal and state funds to meet local needs.
4. Measure and reward outcomes.
5. Embrace a regional mindset. (Ferguson et al., 2020)

She suggested that efforts to modernize federal rural policy would benefit from bringing strategy and coherence, expanding financing for domestic development, and elevating the capacity for building and evaluation.

Ferguson concluded by outlining several strategies for connecting health and development. The first was to adopt asset-based and wealth-building approaches, rather than focusing on deficits. The second was to align health and development strategies, including the required comprehensive economic development strategies and CHNAs. The third was to build partnerships and shared frameworks and vocabulary among rural development hub leaders and population health leaders. The fourth was to build momentum for investing in local people, civic institutions, capacity building, and evaluation. Finally, she suggested joining forces to rewrite the rural narratives to reflect the full diversity and potential of rural people and places.

INNOVATIONS IN SUSTAINING RURAL POPULATION HEALTH

Karen Minyard from the Georgia Health Policy Center discussed insights from the COVID-19 pandemic and explored how to promote financial innovations for sustaining population health. She described a sustainability framework developed by the Georgia Health Policy Center and discussed the mindset required to see the flow of funds in a system and develop financial innovations. Minyard remarked that rural communities are neither monolithic nor completely distinct from one another.

Many subgroups of rural areas share historical, cultural, economic, and geographical commonalities, but they still differ in various ways along the key domains of health care systems, population, environment, infrastructure, and community health status. Infrastructure includes the economy, Internet access, and policy. The health care system includes accessibility, insurance, and the health care workforce. The environment includes climate, housing, exposure, and safety. Population includes culture, demographics, history, and mindsets, she added.

Rural Health Concerns Related to the COVID-19 Pandemic

Minyard explained that at the beginning of the COVID-19 pandemic, the Georgia Health Policy Center asked 200 rural grantees to share concerns regarding rural health. They raised the following key concerns:

- The need for community health workers who could provide social support in the virtual world
- The question of how to deliver effective virtual trainings and conduct effective virtual meetings
- The question of how to handle peer-support services and recovery support related to the opioid epidemic in the pandemic environment
- The need to use telehealth in new ways to meet emerging needs
- The need to adjust approaches to data collection and evaluation during the pandemic
- The need to work with schools to develop strategies to support the community

Minyard described the COVID-19 pandemic as a technological trial by fire, particularly for rural areas. Major challenges that are endemic in rural areas include inconsistent Internet access, lack of cellular service, lack of technology for virtual visits, and discomfort using technology. However, innovation has already emerged from these challenges in rural areas. These include using new telehealth platforms that can function even on low bandwidth Internet connections, the potential integration of COVID-19 measures into electronic health record systems, new strategies to address the health needs in correctional facilities, and the use of school buses to deliver meals. Many of the grantees appreciated having flexibility regarding their HRSA responsibilities in their grants from the Federal Office of Rural Health Policy, because many providers' states had begun to cut their funding. The grantees suggested that going forward, it will be important for them to remain up to date on changing policies, information, and regulations as well as maintaining and expanding telehealth capabilities and developing creative strategies for outreach and connections with clients that incorporate the new measures that were implemented during the pandemic.

Innovations in Sustainability and Financing

Minyard described the framework developed by the Georgia Health Policy Center, which emphasizes the importance of positioning for sustainability. The framework holds that sustainability cannot be established in the short term, leading up to a grant application process. Rather, sustainability is a complex process that must be maintained through strategic vision, collaboration, leadership, relevance and practicality, evaluation and return on investment, communication, efficiency and effectiveness, and capacity. She pointed out that the work described by Bertsch and Barcus included many of these components—including relevance, practicality, evaluation, collaboration, and strategic vision—which will likely contribute to the sustainability of their efforts.

Blueprint for Action to Improve Community Health Through Innovations in Financing

Financing is a critical consideration for sustaining rural population health, said Minyard. Funding sources must be identified within health systems, and implementers must develop innovative strategies to achieve their aims using available funds. In this sense, she added, innovation occurs when the flow of funds is influenced to drive improvements in targeted communities. Such innovations typically involve the application, combination, and creation of financing tools and methods. The Georgia Health Policy Center developed a blueprint for action, which shows how to improve community health through innovative financing (see Figure 5-1).

The blueprint underlines the importance of stewardship and strategy as elements that inform the financing process and how they can be used to answer questions related to funding. Financial instruments can only be implemented after ascertaining how much money is needed initially and annually, the expected returns on investment, and how funds will be administered. She added that finding overlooked sources of funding, such as local governments or banks, requires a broad view of how money flows through public health systems. Focusing only on particular financial instruments is not a substitute for a broad understanding of a system's finances, she noted. Instead, the funding process must be connected to the broader process of innovation. Community collaboratives require an

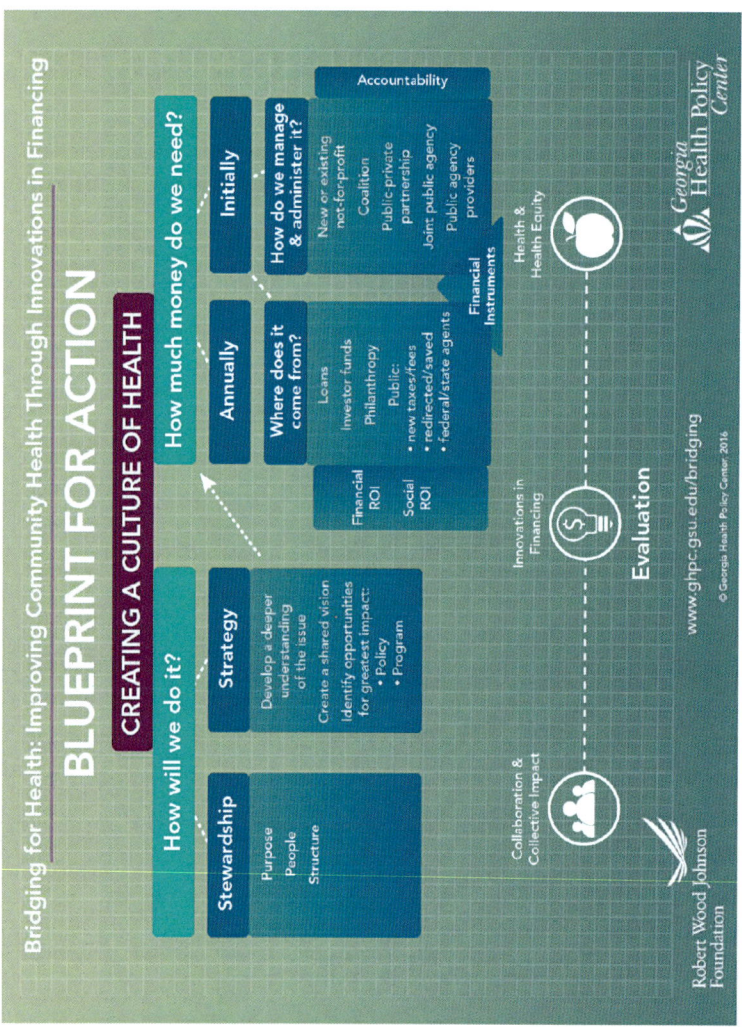

FIGURE 5-1 Blueprint for action for improving community health through innovations in financing.
NOTE: ROI = return on investment.
SOURCES: Minyard presentation, June 25, 2020; www.ghpc.gsu.edu (accessed October 28, 2020).

evolutionary, not revolutionary, approach to financing population health, she added.

Minyard described a cycle of innovation that supported the development of the blueprint for action. The cycle begins with defining and agreeing on the terms and aims of a process, followed by a process of ideation and prototyping that can be used to develop innovations. These prototypes must then be tested and implemented with empathy and an appropriate mindset. The next step is to define and agree on terms for further iterations of the cycle. She shared that seven community collaboratives used this approach to develop a model of local wellness funds, which are vehicles for consolidating all locally available money. For communities to make progress in developing such pooled community wellness funds, questions about sources, uses, and structure need to be answered: (1) Where does the money come from? (2) What will the funds be used for? and (3) How will the funds be managed, administered, and stewarded? She added that maintaining a focus on the financing innovation—not program implementation—is critical but often challenging.

Spurring Innovations in Financing

Minyard remarked that a broader understanding of how money flows through systems requires both an appropriate mindset and open-mindedness. She said these are necessary to see beyond the obvious systemic and financial factors to identify the entire flow of funds. However, all levels of funding are to be seen together to develop innovative financing. She described those with a skill for seeing the flow of funds across a system as "money whisperers," and she asserted that anyone could learn this skill with practice. Money whisperers might see money at the macro (system) level or micro (program) level. She offered two examples of this kind of insight. In one case, a rural banker realized that they could use their bank's money to establish a loan and grant system to accomplish the community's population health goals. In another community, a source of funding was identified within the local government. It had been earmarked to return to the general fund, but because they identified it they were able to divert it to a specific population health project.

Minyard closed by describing several steps to help cultivate the right mindset for innovations in financing. When focusing on population health, thinking should move upstream to look for approaches with the greatest leverage to improve health and well-being. Steps should be taken that also examine the flow of funds, taking care to look in the unlikely places where funds may be flowing. She also suggested building a culture of stewardship and shared collaboration among diverse stakeholder groups. To explore financing vehicles, it is helpful to bear in mind that innovations in funding may include a combination of multiple vehicles to meet the needs of the local context. She suggested looking for intersections of health, money, and partners and encouraging collective investments in health and well-being. These steps should be repeated cyclically to ensure that the innovation cycle continues, Minyard added.

DISCUSSION

Equity in Rural Health

Smart opened the discussion by noting that there are 13 million people of color living in rural America, along with more than 2 million immigrants living in booming immigrant communities across the country. Many of those individuals are not well integrated into the traditional work of nonprofit organizations, institutions, and governments. He asked the panel how to ensure that all individuals in rural communities are incorporated in the works of rural health organizations.

Ferguson replied that a first step is to recognize and acknowledge the existence of racial inequities and other inequities of all kinds. Another step is to expand the understanding of leadership in the context of community-based strategies by bearing in mind that leaders come in all forms. For instance, a mother who is well connected to her community and knows more about the cultural needs and norms of her community might have better community leadership skills than a business executive or elected official. Ferguson added that various approaches can be used to engage the community, such as participatory democracy, to help ensure that decisions made duly reflect a community and its vision. For instance, organizers may choose to provide child care at meetings and choose not to hold meetings at times when only those paid to attend will be able to attend. Ferguson also noted the need to move away from expectations that people should fit within the dominant cultural context and to move toward more openness to different types of norms by adopting a more humble attitude, maintaining an open mind, and asking more questions to learn from the valuable experiences of others.

Barcus added that hospitals also need to maintain a community-centered perspective by meeting people where they are and potentially receiving uncomfortable feedback. She shared an example from a hospital that was conducting a CHNA. The hospital was dedicated to addressing breast cancer in their community, yet data from the community revealed a great burden of prostate cancer among African American men. The hospital's administrators consulted with a local pastor of an African American church, who told them that they should come to the church to encourage men to take action on prostate health, rather than expect those men to attend a seminar on prostate health at the hospital. Minyard commented that not everyone within rural communities holds the same views regarding race and racism, so it is important to be sensitive and responsive to differing viewpoints on complex situations.

Engaging Stakeholders, Changing the Narrative, and Securing Financing

Smart asked the panel to share more insights about garnering financial support for population health efforts, given that population health work is both expensive and lacking a standard funding mechanism. Bertsch suggested engaging with community-based extension offices, for example, and noted that some resources are more accessible through collaboration among providers to seek out different types of available funding. Collaboration can minimize individual responsibility among providers and reduce the financial resources that need to be expended. Ferguson pointed out that the costs of population health are not as expensive as the costs of caring for people who are sick. She suggested shifting the narrative to change policy and make financing available for population health, because most existing funding streams are designated for services rather than health care. Like other infrastructure improvements, financing should be channeled to the upfront costs of ensuring that the necessary population health coordination, strategies, and capacities are put in place to reduce costs in the long term.

Ferguson maintained that federal policy should be aligned with the aims of population health and recognize that population health spending is a long-term investment. Currently, sufficient funding is not available to rural communities to enable them to carry out the needed long-term investments in population health. Piecemeal funding may be available to these communities through various streams, amounting to as much as approximately $100 million, but that does not compare to the approximately $23 to $28 billion spent each year on economic infrastructure investment. She suggested that there is such limited investment in population health because of a misalignment of cultural values and the nature of budgetary systems. Sufficient emphasis has not been placed on the critical role of population health, and budgets are created with a short-term perspective that gives short shrift to the value of long-term investments. Thus, it is necessary to take control of the narrative around health spending and to emphasize the value of prevention in order to bring about real policy changes.

Ferguson suggested leveraging any and all available strategic and funding opportunities in order to make progress toward those immediate aims. Bertsch pointed out the complexities related to the incentives created by value-based approaches to health care. A focus on prevention can disincentivize the provision of services, but, going forward, value can be realized by the wise use of existing resources. Additionally, insurance providers, Medicare, and Medicaid offer payment for the provision of preventive services, said Bertsch.

Making the Case for Philanthropic Spending in Rural Population Health

Smart asked why philanthropists ought to invest in rural population health. Ferguson replied that the current model of rural health care is not workable. Indicators of health status and health outcomes are worsening, and rural hospitals are closing, so rural health warrants a radical systemwide transformation. This need creates an opportunity for philanthropic organizations to be impactful; impact is often a key criterion for philanthropic organizations seeking opportunities to invest. The rural health space is open to creative, risk-taking, and innovative approaches to realizing transformations. Ferguson remarked that philanthropists can help "blaze a trail" toward new models of population health, which governments and others may subsequently follow, because philanthropists are uniquely suited to take on the risk of investing in population health while also helping to drive change at the local level.

Panel Reflections

Smart invited the panel to give their final reflections on the session. Bertsch remarked on the importance of convening a diversity of expertise to address the challenges of population health. Diversity is a key aspect of community collaboration—including racial diversity and diversity in the provision of services—thus bringing more stakeholders to the table improves outcomes for all. Barcus emphasized the value of collaboration and engaging all stakeholders, such as art communities, theater and music communities, businesses, churches, and any other community groups that are concerned about health. Ferguson highlighted the need to bridge community economic development and health and the need to develop intellectual frameworks and language that enable individuals working on the ground to recognize that they are partners and allies in this work. Those working in health care, water infrastructure, and business development are all working to create more and better opportunities for better health outcomes for rural communities.

Ferguson suggested that by collaborating across geographies and industries, stakeholders can articulate a vision for the future of rural communities. Minyard underscored the importance of seeing how money flows through systems, leveraging the skills of "money whisperers" to serve as leaders in their communities or regions, and organizing funding streams in a way that supports population health. In closing, Smart remarked that the best rural philanthropic work often incorporates ideas raised by the panelists, including multidisciplinary community partnering. He suggested that rural settings should be considered as *places* first, rather than as the locus of a particular set of issues.

6

Rural Health Policy

The workshop's session on rural health policy introduced a variety of U.S. federal policies affecting rural health. It featured presentations on shifting rural health policy and practice toward value-based care, strategies for engaging health care providers to confront the health care crisis in rural America, the structure and function of tribal rural health policy, and the implications for rural health of the congressional response to the coronavirus disease 2019 (COVID-19) pandemic. Karen Murphy, chief innovation officer at The Steele Institute for Health Innovation at Geisinger Health, moderated the session.

SHIFTING RURAL HEALTH POLICY AND PRACTICE TOWARD VALUE-BASED CARE

Tim Putnam, president and chief executive officer (CEO) of Margaret Mary Health in Indiana, discussed how rural health organizations focus on population health, form collaborative partnerships, and create policy and practices centered on prevention and primary care. He described how a rural hospital can shift from focusing on medical interventions to prioritizing prevention and population health using the example of Margaret Mary Health, a small community hospital in Batesville, Indiana (see Box 6-1). He shared lessons his institution has learned in making this transition, as well as how the hospital has been affected by, and has responded to, the COVID-19 pandemic. He also highlighted the value of prevention efforts and the role of rural hospitals in this work.

> **BOX 6-1**
> **Margaret Mary Health**
>
> Margaret Mary Health is a small community hospital in Batesville, Indiana, formed in 1932. Three years into the Great Depression, the community assessed how to help one another, especially those most in need, and they decided to create a hospital. The hospital's mission is "to be the best health care provider for our communities where people choose to come for services; where physicians choose to practice; and where team members choose to work." The institution's core values are innovation, collaboration, accountability, respect, and excellence. Margaret Mary Health is a critical access hospital, which is the designation used for rural facilities with 25 beds or less. Located about 1 hour from both Indianapolis and Cincinnati, it is 1 of approximately 1,300 critical access hospitals in the country. Margaret Mary Health employs nearly 800 people; annually, it has about 20,000 emergency room visits, 2,000 inpatient admissions, and approximately 500 babies delivered.
>
> SOURCE: Putnam presentation, June 25, 2020.

Rural health care has been and will continue to be the leader in population health, Putnam said. By nature, rural physicians focus on primary care and prevention, which includes addressing social determinants of health (SDOH). He suggested that small rural communities are microcosms of health care delivery and that rural models prioritizing prevention and primary care can be highly effective. The mission of Margaret Mary Health—like many rural hospitals—is to focus on improving the health of community members, which is aligned with the aims of population health to make populations healthier.

Transitioning to Population Health and Value-Based Care in a Rural Hospital

Putnam explained that Margaret Mary Health began transitioning to a focus on population health approximately 7 years ago in order to better serve its community by keeping people healthier. This transition was catalyzed in part by the hospital board's realization that the hospital was neither paid nor incentivized to focus on prevention and control of chronic conditions, such as diabetes. The board decided to make the changes necessary to transition to value-based care and focus on delivering population health services to their community, especially primary care. This transition required establishing multiple new partnerships and coordinating with other rural community health systems. Putnam said the hospital initially considered becoming an accountable care organization (ACO) as the most viable solution, but like most rural hospitals, it did not have the adequate population size to meet the 5,000 Medicare beneficiary minimum required to participate in an ACO. Instead, Margaret Mary Health joined with nine other hospitals in California, Michigan, Oklahoma, and Texas to form the first national rural ACO. This union allowed the hospitals to reach the ACO minimum threshold of 5,000 Medicare beneficiaries. This partnership has created a collaborative effect in improving health care, Putnam noted. When hospitals create partnerships like this, each hospital can share its successes and failures with the others. He added that unlike the competitive relationships between some urban hospitals, rural hospitals tend to be less competitive and more supportive in wanting other rural hospitals to be effective and successful, and to have good outcomes.

Putnam described several lessons learned during Margaret Mary Health's transition to a focus on population health. Initially, the institution adopted a "hospital perspective" in focusing 80–90 percent of its health care costs on 10–20 percent of its patients (e.g., people with severe chronic conditions). Hospital management soon realized the need to shift from a predominant focus on high-end patients to a greater focus on keeping people healthy. Margaret Mary Health engaged with primary care physicians to gain insights about how to focus on prevention, finding that they needed to get closer to patients and learn how their lifestyles and home life related to health. This can allow for strategies to address SDOH and encourage people to have annual wellness visits. Hospital management also learned that care coordinators can be instrumental in this effort, because physicians trust the care coordinators and convey that trust to patients. Putnam suggested that this type of shift from a "hospital focus" toward emphasizing primary and preventive care for communities enables rural health systems to lead the effort in population health.

Data are a core component of delivering population health services effectively, said Putnam. Being part of an ACO enables health systems to request Medicare claims information about patients, which provides a "treasure trove" of data that make it possible to build the knowledge base and avoid guesswork. To illustrate, he described a physician whose patients' pharmaceutical costs were 20 percent higher than those of other physicians' patients. She was perplexed because she was prescribing the same medications as her colleagues. In analyzing the data, they found that her patients' emergency department (ED) costs were much lower, indicating that the decrease in ED visits and the higher prescription expenditures were the result of that physician's efforts to motivate her patients to take their medications as prescribed without lapses between refills.

Effect of COVID-19 in a Rural Hospital

Putnam used the experience of Margaret Mary Health to describe the effect of COVID-19 on rural hospitals early in the pandemic (Goodnough, 2020). Margaret Mary Health treated its first patient with COVID-19 on March 13, 2020, and had to adapt quickly as the hospital exceeded regular capacity when the hospital's service area was hit hard by the virus early on, causing a huge increase in patient load. Typically, the hospital's inpatient services account for about 20 percent of care provision and outpatient services account for 80 percent. As more patients with COVID-19 crashed within hours of arrival at the hospital, this ratio shifted to 20 percent outpatient services and 200 percent inpatient services. Putnam said the transition to value-based care was helpful during the COVID-19 response as it allowed them to simultaneously meet the needs of patients with COVID-19 as well as the needs of their existing 2,000 ACO patients. With care coordinators in physician offices already in place, a structure existed for meeting the needs of regular patients through these trusted professionals. Many of the patients with COVID-19 were receiving primary care services from Margaret Mary Health, so the hospital had prior knowledge about their medical histories. Furthermore, Putnam said some of the patients most vulnerable to COVID-19—such as those with diabetes, high blood pressure, chronic obstructive pulmonary disease, and congestive heart failure—already had those chronic conditions under control prior to the pandemic. Putnam suggested that having a healthy population—in this case, a result of the shift in focus to population health—was a major boon to the COVID-19 response at Margaret Mary Health.

Toward Value-Based Care

Putnam remarked on how rural health systems can lead the way in the shift to value-based care moving forward. Although "an ounce of prevention is worth a pound of cure," the axiom of Benjamin Franklin, the current reimbursement models for health care are focused on paying for and incentivizing cures rather than prevention. He noted that rural health care providers are able to witness the positive effects of prevention because of their close relationships with patients in their small communities. Moving forward, Margaret Mary Health is emphasizing annual wellness visits so patients see their physicians *before* they are sick. This is a challenge, as many people do not see the value of wellness visits, but the care coordinators and nurses in the system are helping patients understand that wellness visits—which may include screenings, prevention efforts, and immunizations—are a way of keeping people healthy.

Putnam said the rural setting is a microcosm of the world and that it is well suited for prevention work. Rural health systems are small, and the chief of staff is typically a primary care physician rather than the cardiovascular surgeons or high-end researchers who typically hold those types of positions in urban hospitals. The hospital CEOs and other leaders in rural health systems meet on a regular basis to connect with one another. The shared mission is to keep their communities healthier, so prevention is a priority from the start. In an urban setting, hospital board meetings may address topics such as the latest cancer proton beam therapy or the transplant program. In contrast, rural boards of directors focus on how to offer basic services to keep patients healthy. Putnam emphasized that these features of rural health settings are at the core of successful population health efforts. He noted that the same types of shifts in focus toward prevention and primary care efforts that were undertaken at Margaret Mary Health are also occurring in other small communities across the country, which will contribute to the success of broader population health efforts.

ENGAGING HEALTH CARE PROVIDERS TO CONFRONT RURAL AMERICA'S HEALTH CARE CRISIS

Keith Mueller is a Gerhard Hartman professor and head of the Department of Health Management and Policy from The University of Iowa and director of the Rural Policy Research Institute Center for Rural Policy Analysis. He provided an overview of recommendations from a report prepared by the Rural Health Task Force of the Bipartisan Policy Center (BPC)—*Confronting Rural America's Healthcare Crisis*.[1] These recommendations address issues such as short-term financial stabilization, long-term financial sustainability, workforce shortages, infrastructure needs, and the development of new models of service financing and delivery. The recommendations include measures to (1) strengthen financial stability and sustainability; (2) increase flexibility in using resources, including the health care workforce; (3) create new models of financing and delivering services; and (4) improve health infrastructure. The task force included an array of rural health experts, such as rural health policy experts, health care systems leaders, and clinical practitioners. The report was developed via a series of roundtable discussions featuring stakeholder presentations, site visits, and work with congressional staff.

---

[1] The report is available at https://bipartisanpolicy.org/report/confronting-rural-americas-health-care-crisis (accessed September 9, 2020).

Strategies to Engage Health Care Providers in Population Health

In his presentation, Mueller focused on the report's recommendations that he described as essential to engaging health care providers in population health, including short- and long-term financial stability, flexibility in resource use and incentives, and infrastructure support.

Short-Term Financial Stability

Stabilizing health care delivery in rural America is the first step in engaging providers in population health, said Mueller. Stabilization efforts involve addressing short-term circumstances for rural hospitals. One of the report's recommendation to improve hospitals' short-term financial stability is relief from Medicare sequestration payment reductions for rural hospitals. Sequestration relief was put in place for the duration of the COVID-19 pandemic,[2] and the task force recommends that this be extended through the year 2023. In addition, the group advised increasing payments to critical access hospitals (CAHs) by 3 percent. Other recommendations pertain to the criteria for designating rural health care facilities: reestablish the "CAH necessary provider" designation,[3] and make permanent both the Medicare-dependent hospital designation and the low-volume adjustment hospital designation, rather than being subject to periodic renewals. Beyond hospitals, the task force also made recommendations regarding other providers, added Mueller. These include (1) paying rural clinicians reporting data under the Quality Payment Program, (2) extending bonus payments for new advanced alternative model participants, and (3) leveraging patient engagement incentives to decrease rural bypass and incentivize local care utilization.

Long-Term Financial Sustainability

The BPC Rural Health Task Force made a separate set of recommendations for improving long-term financial stability, said Mueller. For example, grants and loans for capital infrastructure could enable the maintenance of service lines and improve both structural safety and

---

[2] Sequestration is the automatic reduction (i.e., cancellation) of certain federal spending, generally by a uniform percentage. The sequester is a budget enforcement tool that was established by Congress in the Balanced Budget and Emergency Deficit Control Act of 1985 (BBEDCA, also known as the Gramm-Rudman-Hollings Act; P.L. 99-177, as amended). See https://crsreports.congress.gov/product/pdf/R/R45106 (accessed October 20, 2020).

[3] Mueller noted that in the early years of the CAH program, states were able to designate facilities as CAH even if they did not meet federally designated CAH criteria, such as being at least 35 miles from another hospital.

patient safety. Capital infrastructure could also include converting facilities from the classic inpatient model into alternatives featuring increased outpatient services. Another recommendation was to enact payment reforms that would stabilize rural health clinics and expand access to advanced practice clinician services in these rural clinics. Mueller said he believed that certain existing Medicare-related regulations inhibit the success of rural health clinics and should be removed.

The task force also recommended that the Medicare-capped reimbursement rate for physician-owned rural health clinics should be increased. Currently, the physician-owned clinic reimbursement rate is lower than that for hospital-owned rural health clinics. It was recommended that enrolled ACO beneficiaries should be excluded when determining regional benchmarks in rural areas. Many of the beneficiaries in rural areas are ACO-attributed lives, and the shared savings of ACOs drive down expenditures for these individuals. Therefore, Mueller suggested that these beneficiaries not be accounted for in benchmarks, because doing so would affect the ability to generate shared savings in subsequent years. The shared savings of ACOs can be assessed based on benchmarks derived from data on previous practices, he added.

Flexibility in Resource Use

Flexibility in resource use—including human resources—is central to engaging providers in population health, said Mueller. He highlighted several of the task force's recommendations that allow for greater flexibility in using resources. For example, it recommended that rules around colocation or shared space arrangements should be clarified to enable rural hospitals to partner more effectively with other health care organizations. It also recommended that advanced practice clinicians should be allowed to work up to their state's scope of practice in rural health clinics. Similarly, the task force recommended removing regulatory and legislative barriers that prevent nonphysician providers from practicing at the top of their license. Mueller noted that steps have been taken during the COVID-19 pandemic to remove these restrictions and suggested that this flexibility be extended beyond the pandemic. Billing regulations currently prohibit Medicare beneficiaries from receiving multiple same-day services within the same specialty, which limits a provider to payment for one service per day. Therefore, the task force recommended exempting rural Medicare beneficiaries from this prohibition to allow greater flexibility for rural providers.

Incentives and Flexibility

Mueller noted that the task force emphasized the need for hospital transformation plans that allow facilities in rural areas to reflect the needs of their service areas more appropriately. Thus, it recommended putting in place incentives for rural facilities and communities that develop hospital transformation plans. The task force also suggested moving toward three alternative models of financing. The first is a new "rural and emergency outpatient hospital" designation that would include cost-based reimbursement. Moving away from inpatient-centered care, this designation would be an option for communities whose needs are largely emergency and outpatient care.[4] The second model would establish an Extended Rural Services Program. To support communities where hospital-level services become unavailable because of hospital closures or reductions in capacity, this program would allow federally qualified health centers (FQHCs) and rural health clinics to offer hospital-level services that would otherwise be unavailable. The third is a multipayer global budget model that would shift the focus from hospital expenditures to total expenditures. Global budget models are currently being demonstrated in Pennsylvania, and one is operating in its second generation in Maryland. The task force also recommended decreasing participation thresholds for rural providers for all these alternative payment models, as well as rural health clinics and FQHCs, added Mueller. Program participation criteria are often biased toward larger populations, so alternative payment models for smaller population sizes are needed for rural areas.

Infrastructure Support

Mueller explained that the task force made an additional set of longer-term recommendations to address infrastructure support. The need for broadband services in rural areas has gained attention during the pandemic, leading to legislation being passed to extend and augment current provisions. The task force recommended prioritizing the connection of rural areas with broadband through anchor institutions and direct-to-home services, as well as ensuring effective implementation of the Broadband Deployment Accuracy and Technological Availability Act.[5] They recommended that telehealth service use could be supported

---

[4] Mueller noted that this model is included in legislation co-sponsored by Senator Chuck Grassley of Iowa, who served as a member of the Honorary Congressional Task Force on Rural Health that collaborated with the BPC Rural Health Task force.

[5] More information about the Broadband Deployment Accuracy and Technological Availability Act is available at https://www.congress.gov/bill/116th-congress/house-bill/4229/text (accessed September 9, 2020).

by changes in payment policies, provider eligibility, location of sites of service, and eligible services. In response to COVID-19, all of these issues were included in legislation and regulatory changes. However, those provisions are time limited and will expire with the public health emergency. Mueller suggested that the temporary changes that worked effectively should be extended beyond the pandemic.

Additional Recommendations Related to Population Health

Mueller outlined several other recommendations related to population health made by the task force:

- Increase the number of rural-specific Center for Medicare & Medicaid Innovation demonstrations and expedite the expansion of promising models to the national level.
- Reduce the administrative burden on rural providers by using readily available claims data for quality performance.
- Improve access to quality maternal care in rural areas (four specific recommendations, including increasing the funding for maternal health training programs for primary care providers).
- Improve use of the currently available workforce (five specific recommendations, including expanding reimbursement to additional provider types and extending Medicare-covered status to additional mental health providers).
- Strengthen the Health Resources and Services Administration (HRSA) rural workforce programs (two specific recommendations).
- Expand federal rural workforce recruitment and retention initiatives (four specific recommendations).
- Authorize licensed clinicians to provide interstate services to Medicare beneficiaries.[6]
- Direct The Office of the National Coordinator for Health Information Technology to prioritize rural-specific training curricula for the health information technology workforce.

Conditions for Addressing Population Health

Mueller concluded by listing a set of necessary conditions to address population health from his perspective. These conditions include a financially secure delivery system with predictable financial resources and payment systems that support engagement in community-driven population

---

[6] Mueller noted that this has been enacted temporarily in response to the COVID-19 pandemic.

health programming. He called for flexibility in how health systems are built and restructured through transformation plans. Flexibility is also needed in how professionals practice and how patients interact with a range of professionals. Finally, Mueller suggested that the BPC Task Force recommendations are building blocks for moving toward population health.

TRIBAL RURAL HEALTH POLICY

Benjamin Smith, deputy director for intergovernmental affairs for the Indian Health Service (IHS), provided an overview of the origin of IHS and its role in health policy development for American Indians and Alaska Natives. He described the breadth of facilities within IHS and outlined some of the current health challenges faced by American Indians. He also discussed the effect of the Indian Health Care Improvement Act (IHCIA) on current and future policy decisions related to the health of American Indians and Alaska Natives.

Smith is a member of the Navajo Nation and grew up on the Navajo Reservation in a rural, remote area. He is a second-generation federal employee within IHS, as his father was an IHS physician. Therefore, he has the dual perspective of witnessing firsthand the provision of federal services to American Indians and understanding how policy decisions are made within the federal government. He explained that IHS is committed to providing quality health care consistent with statutory authorities and the government-to-government relationship of the United States with American Indians and Alaska Natives. Serving members of 574 federally recognized tribes, IHS is a comprehensive health service delivery system for approximately 2.6 million individuals. IHS has an annual budget appropriation of approximately $6 billion and employs more than 15,300 people, including nurses, physicians, pharmacists, sanitarians,[7] physician assistants, and dentists.

History of the Indian Health Service

To provide historical context, Smith traced the origins of what would later become IHS back to the 18th and 19th centuries. During that time, the U.S. government entered into treaties with American Indians and

---

[7] A sanitarian is an investigator of health and safety within an environment. This may be the workplace, food preparation facilities, industrial producers, or even the general environment. Sanitarians not only enforce health and safety regulation, but they also identify risk factors between people and in specific spaces. See https://www.careersinpublichealth.net/careers/sanitarian (accessed October 20, 2020).

Alaska Natives. In trading land for education, health care, and other services, a relationship was formed between the U.S. government and American Indians and Alaska Natives that required a series of policies to manage this partnership. Beginning in the early 1800s, the Administration of Indian Affairs was located in the Department of War. He noted that this may seem an unusual location for an organization focused on government-to-government relationships. However, as the United States was expanding westward, many health care services were located in military forts providing episodic care. The Department of War was therefore seen as the most effective department for housing the Administration of Indian Affairs and responding to the health care needs of American Indians and Alaska Natives. In 1849, oversight and administration of Indian health was transferred from the Department of War to the civilian Bureau of Indian Affairs located within the Department of the Interior. Congress first appropriated funding specifically for health services to Indians in 1911 in the amount of $40,000, which would be approximately $1 million today. Milestone legislation came in 1921 with the Snyder Act, which defined the U.S. government's responsibility for American Indian health care. IHS continues to work off the Snyder Act today, in addition to other subsequent milestones.

Smith explained that IHS was formally established by law through the Transfer Act of 1955, which transferred all health facilities operated by the Bureau of Indian Affairs—many of which were in schools or health centers attached to schools—to what is now called the Department of Health and Human Services (HHS). Around that time, the Committee on Appropriations of the House of Representatives directed the U.S. Public Health Service to conduct a comprehensive survey of the status of Indian health in general and report the results to Congress. Published in 1957, this report is commonly referred to as the Gold Book (owing to the color of its cover) and included several notable conclusions, said Smith. First, it found that a substantial federal Indian health program is required. Next, community resources should be developed in cooperation with the American Indian and Alaska Native communities on a reservation-by-reservation basis. Third, federal Indian health programs should be planned in each community and services made available to Indians under state and local programs. Finally, efforts should be made to recognize the obligations and responsibilities to Indian residents on a nondiscriminatory basis from the state and local communities.

Smith emphasized the ramifications of these findings. With 574 federally recognized tribes having government-to-government relationships, developing policy addressing all of these findings is no easy task. Therefore, the Gold Book led to other key legislative efforts, such as the Indian Sanitation Facilities Act. Enacted by Congress in 1959, this legislation expanded the Snyder Act and the Transfer Act to include sanitation facilities and services as part of the health care services provided to American Indians. Sanitation construction projects, environmental health programs, and hospital and health clinic construction became public services offered by IHS. Smith noted that water access continues to be a challenge for many American Indian and Alaska Native communities.

Throughout much of the 20th century, federal tribal policy took a "termination" or "assimilation" approach in trying to bring rural communities into urban health centers, Smith said. While each of the federally recognized American Indian and Alaska Native tribes was to have a government-to-government political relationship with the United States, prior federal policies of relocation and assimilation resulted in a large population of native peoples residing in urban centers. In the 1970s, a dramatic policy shift took place, moving from termination to self-determination. The Indian Self-Determination and Education Assistance Act of 1975 authorized government agencies to make grants directly to federally recognized tribes, who then had authority over how they administered the funds. This renewed the government-to-government relationship the U.S. government has with each individual tribe. In 1976, the Indian Healthcare Improvement Act was first enacted, expanding the types of services IHS could provide.

The legislation of the 1970s brought about a new contracting mechanism, noted Smith. Rather than being regulated by the Federal Acquisition Regulations or by the rules and regulations of grants or cooperative agreements, it is a unique contracting mechanism in which the federal government transfers program service functions and activities directly to American Indians and Alaska Natives. This contracting method continues to be reflected in today's IHS through service delivery mechanisms described in the next section.

Indian Health Service Delivery Mechanisms

Smith described three types of service delivery mechanisms available for American Indians and Alaska Natives to choose from. The first is direct service provision from the federal government. The next option is for a tribe or tribal organization to exercise self-governance authority under the Indian Self-Determination and Education Assistance Act in contracting health care programs from the government and operating them tribally at the local level. Norton Sound Health Corporation Hospital is one such facility, operated and managed in Alaska by the Alaska Natives. Some benefits of this option include added flexibility in redesigning programs and the ability to retarget funds to meet health care needs within that local community, he said. The third delivery mechanism is an option for meeting the needs of the large population of American Indians and Alaska Natives residing in urban settings. This involves contracting with nonprofit organizations and nongovernmental, urban Indian organizations. The Indian Healthcare Improvement Act authorized IHS's Urban Indian Health Program and funds 41 urban-centered, nonprofit organizations nationwide.[8]

IHS has a diverse range of health care facilities across the United States that use these three delivery mechanisms, said Smith. These facilities include those directly operated by IHS, tribal health programs, and the urban-centered organizations. With hospitals, health care centers, clinics, health stations, school health centers, and youth regional treatment centers, great variety exists in IHS-affiliated facilities. The majority of facilities are tribal health programs, meaning a tribe or tribal organization operates the facility pursuant to the Indian Self-Determination and Education Assistance Act. This is evident in the state of Alaska, which is home to more than 200 federally recognized Alaska Native villages. Alaska has 58 tribal health centers, 160 tribal community health clinics, and 6 tribally operated hospitals.[9] Smith noted that since populations can be very small, village clinics are important. Furthermore, he pointed out that at these smaller facilities, health objectives at the local level are targeted in decision making and policy setting within a tribal government.

Community Health Representatives Program

Another long-standing aspect of rural health care provision to American Indians and Alaska Natives is community outreach, Smith said. In response to the needs expressed by tribal governments, organizations, and IHS, Congress established an outreach program in 1968. The Community Health Representatives (CHR) program was designed to bridge the gap between patients in the community and health care facilities providing care.[10] Predating the Indian Self-Determination and Education Assistance Act, the CHR program was the first formal assumption of an IHS-supported program by an Indian tribe. Smith suggested that rural health can be conceptualized as community members responding

---

[8] More information about the geographic location of these health facilities and the types of programs they offer is available at https://www.ihs.gov/locations (accessed September 9, 2020).

[9] More information about IHS in Alaska is available at https://www.ihs.gov/alaska (accessed September 9, 2020).

[10] More information about the CHR program is available at https://www.ihs.gov/chr (accessed September 9, 2020) and https://www.ihs.gov/ihm/pc/part-3/p3c16/#3-16.3C (accessed September 9, 2020).

to health care needs and using their own language to translate needs and services in a culturally appropriate and acceptable way.

Challenges Faced by the Indian Health Service

Smith remarked that tribal governments and IHS face great health challenges, like much of the rural United States. For example, life expectancy is substantially shorter for American Indians and Alaska Natives (at 4.4 years less) than the average for the entire U.S. population.[11] Funding is a barrier, as reflected in data from the National Congress of American Indians and the National Indian Health Board indicating that per capita expenditures are lower for IHS than for other groups. IHS uses a pricing model called the Federal Disparity Index to compare IHS funding for medical services with that of the Federal Employees Health Plan.[12] This index shows that current funding meets 48.6 percent of the need, Smith said, and Congress appropriates less than half of what IHS requires to carry out its statutory authorities each year. Remote locations and government hiring freezes make workforce recruitment and retention difficult. Furthermore, Smith noted challenges related to government parity in salary and leave. Aging facilities and equipment are issues, with outdated main facilities held over from the transfer from the Department of the Interior and equipment shortages in hospitals, clinics, and service units. This also affects recruitment and retention, as candidates who have just completed years of training and education may not be familiar with the outdated equipment still used in some IHS facilities. Smith added that IHS is working toward electronic health record (EHR) modernization, but it continues to face health information technology challenges related to data security and lack of infrastructure in rural sites.

Policy Ramifications of the Indian Health Care Improvement Act

Smith said that the IHCIA,[13] made permanent with the passage of the Patient Protection and Affordable Care Act of 2010, covers a number of topics and underscores federal policy related to Indian health. It sets the goal of ensuring the highest possible health status for American Indians and Alaska Natives, benchmarked with the objectives of the

---

[11] Life Expectancy American Indians and Alaska Natives Data Years 2007–2009. See https://www.ihs.gov/sites/dps/themes/responsive2017/display_objects/documents/LifeExpectancy2007-09ReportMemo.pdf (accessed October 26, 2020).

[12] More information about the Federal Disparity Index is available at https://www.ihs.gov/fdi (accessed September 9, 2020).

[13] More information about the IHCIA is available at https://www.ihs.gov/ihcia (accessed September 9, 2020).

federal Healthy People initiative. He noted that IHS has been working to update those objectives to include the rural component, because tribes and tribal organizations fall into this category. He said that American Indian participation has been ensured and maximized by the IHCIA, which defined a new form of communication through tribal consultation and conferral with urban Indian organizations. When the federal government sets policy, the process needs to include tribal and urban partners. Smith said that the IHCIA sets forth objectives for health professionals, uses a government-to-government relationship, and provides the funding necessary for facilities operated both by the Indian Health Service and by tribes. Smith emphasized that as tribes set policies in the future, it is important that the federal government underscore its commitment to providing access to health care to American Indians and Alaska Natives, as established by treaties and within the bounds and scopes of the laws that set forth their authorities.

CONGRESSIONAL RESPONSE TO COVID-19 FOR RURAL AMERICA

Kate Cassling, director of the BPC Action and Bipartisan Policy Center, described the four COVID-19 pandemic response bills passed by Congress between March 6 and April 26, 2020: the Coronavirus Preparedness and Response Supplemental Appropriations Act; the Family First Coronavirus Response Act; the Coronavirus Aid, Relief, and Economic Security (CARES) Act; and the Paycheck Protection Program and Health Care Enhancement Act. She highlighted major components of the legislation, with an emphasis on provisions related to health care and ramifications for rural providers. A discussion of future pandemic legislation ended the presentation.

Coronavirus Preparedness and Response Supplemental Appropriations Act

Cassling explained that the Coronavirus Preparedness and Response Supplemental Appropriations Act (H.R. 6074)[14] was the first bill passed in response to the COVID-19 pandemic. Enacted into law on March 6, 2020, it allocated $7.8 billion to a variety of agencies addressing pandemic-related issues such as health problems and economic challenges. Funding included $2.2 billion to the Centers for Disease Control and Prevention

---

[14] More information about the Coronavirus Preparedness and Response Supplemental Appropriations Act is available at https://www.congress.gov/bill/116th-congress/house-bill/6074 (accessed September 9, 2020).

(CDC), $836 million for the National Institute of Allergy and Infectious Diseases, $61 million for the Food and Drug Administration, and $20 million for disaster loans via the Small Business Administration (SBA). The Public Health and Social Services Emergency Fund received $3.1 billion with this measure, including $100 million for HRSA for grants under the Health Centers Program.

Families First Coronavirus Response Act

Given the rapid deterioration of the health situation and the problematic nature of the economic situation in the early phases of the COVID-19 pandemic, Congress quickly realized further support was needed, said Cassling. On March 18, 2020, the Families First Coronavirus Response Act (H.R. 6201)[15] was signed into law, providing an additional $3.47 billion in funding. A large portion of this support was dedicated to maintaining access to nutrition services that are critical for many people in both urban and rural environments, such as the Supplemental Nutrition Assistance Program; the Special Supplemental Nutrition Program for Women, Infants, and Children; and the Emergency Food Assistance Program. It also allocated an additional $1 billion to the Public Health and Social Services Emergency Fund specifically to help health care providers cover the cost of COVID-19 testing for the uninsured. Furthermore, the bill provided a temporary increase in the federal match for Medicaid, expanded access to paid sick leave, and required that COVID-19 testing and related services be covered without cost-sharing across payers such as Medicare, Medicaid, and private insurance.

Coronavirus Aid, Relief, and Economic Security Act

Signed into law on March 27, 2020, as the largest stimulus bill in U.S. history, the CARES Act (S. 3548)[16] allocated more than $2 trillion for economic relief in the wake of the pandemic. Cassling remarked that the speed with which this large spending bill passed with bipartisan support is rare, indicating the importance of the pandemic-related problems and profound concern on the part of members of Congress. She added that the bill touched every part of the economy and the health care industry. The CARES Act included economic measures, such as expanding

---

[15] More information about the Families First Coronavirus Response Act is available at https://www.congress.gov/bill/116th-congress/house-bill/6201 (accessed September 9, 2020).

[16] More information about the CARES Act is available at https://www.congress.gov/bill/116th-congress/senate-bill/3548 (accessed September 21, 2021) and https://home.treasury.gov/policy-issues/cares (accessed September 9, 2020).

unemployment insurance with a $600 per week benefit increase. Cassling noted the July 2020 expiration date for this benefit has become a focus of conversations around needed future steps should economic conditions not improve. Also included in the CARES Act were recovery rebates of $1,200 issued to many Americans below an income cap. State and local governments received $150 billion in funding, and $500 billion was allocated to mid-sized and large businesses. Additionally, this legislation created the Paycheck Protection Program (PPP) through SBA, which provided loans to small businesses with fewer than 500 employees, including rural health providers. Although $350 billion was initially allocated to PPP, there were some early implementation difficulties. Cassling commented that challenges will arise any time a bureaucracy is tasked with pushing out large amounts of money in a short amount of time, but, in this case, rural health providers, "mom and pop" business owners, and minority-owned businesses struggled to access the first round of PPP funding. Since then, the Department of the Treasury, SBA, and Congress have taken steps to address this issue, making it easier for rural providers and others to access PPP loans, added Cassling.

CARES Act Funding for Rural Providers

Cassling explained that many rural health care providers received some type of financial support via the CARES Act because it included numerous provisions related to health care. An allocation of $100 billion was designated for hospitals, physician practices, and other health care providers. This funding was two-fold: first, to compensate for revenue lost to canceled elective procedures, and second, to cover the increased costs of pandemic-related needs such as personal protective equipment (PPE), testing supplies, and emergency operations. Cassling said HHS was balancing between the need to transfer large amounts of money quickly on the one hand, and ensuring that funds are sent to appropriate recipients on the other. Initially, HHS used past Medicare payments to determine amounts sent to individual providers. This worked well for some providers, but the method was problematic for children's hospitals and facilities that traditionally relied on Medicaid payments. Over time, HHS determined that funding set-asides were needed to ensure that particular populations were not overlooked. To that end, HHS set aside $10 billion specifically for rural providers.

Additional measures for economic stability include the suspension of the 2 percent Medicare sequester until December 31, 2020, which was referenced early by Mueller. A 20 percent Medicare add-on payment was provided for treating COVID-19 patients. The CARES Act also expanded the Medicare Accelerated Payments Program, which provides upfront loans for providers based on what future Medicare payments are expected to be. Cassling said this was rolled out fairly smoothly, yet it was suspended by HHS because of its effect on the Medicare trust fund. She said that some rural providers report that they cannot necessarily repay these loans under current circumstances, however. This has led to bipartisan conversations at the federal level about how to adjust repayment for those loans, whether by lowering interest rates, changing the payment schedule, or forgiving the loans entirely. In spite of bipartisan support, Cassling stated that the major challenge to adjusting loan repayment is funding, given the state of the Medicare trust fund and issues with solvency. The CARES Act also provided grant funding, including $1.32 billion for community health centers and $180 million in HRSA grants designated specifically for strengthening telehealth and rural community health.

Additional CARES Health Provisions

Cassling noted that the CARES Act includes additional provisions regarding extending health care programs, the health care workforce, and telehealth access. "Health extenders" are a group of provisions extending funding for a collective of health care programs such as the Community Health Centers Fund, the National Health Service Corps, and the Teaching Health Centers Graduate Medical Education program. Because of ongoing debate about how to fund health extenders, they were set to expire in May 2020. COVID-19 raised concerns about ending health programs during a pandemic, thus the CARES Act reauthorized the health extenders through November 30, 2020. The legislation also includes several provisions to meet the increased demand for health care services, such as immunity from malpractice lawsuits to health care professionals who volunteer to provide medical care during the pandemic. It also authorized the reassignment of National Health Service Corps providers to respond to COVID-19 and established a Ready Reserve Corps of trained doctors and nurses to respond to this pandemic as well as future health emergencies.

Cassling stated that a series of governmental actions in response to COVID-19, such as appropriations bills and regulatory changes, have dramatically increased access to telehealth services. The CARES Act allowed FQHCs and rural health clinics to provide telehealth services to Medicare patients in their homes, which opened the door to phone-based services for patients who do not have high-speed Internet access. HRSA telehealth grant programs were expanded to specifically help providers set up this service and obtain the tools and technical assistance needed to use it. The CARES Act also included funding for broadband investment, providing $125 million to the Rural Utilities Service. Cassling contended that the broadband investment gap is in the billions, rather than the millions, but he said this step recognized that providing telehealth in rural communities requires access to high-speed Internet. She continued that the U.S. administration has pushed for reimbursement parity and has increased the number of people eligible for various types of telehealth programs. Moving forward, she predicted a continued relaxing of telehealth regulations that will be of particular benefit to rural health communities contending with access issues.

Paycheck Protection Program and Health Care Enhancement Act

Cassling described the fourth bill in response to COVID-19—the PPP and Health Care Enhancement Act (H.R. 266). Passed on April 26, 2020, the legislation allocated $500 billion in additional funding and addressed some technical problems in the CARES Act. As it went into law only 1 month after the $2 trillion CARES Act, the need for this bill reflects the high level of challenges brought on by the pandemic. The bulk of funding, $321 billion, was for the PPP, which extends to rural employers with fewer than 500 employees. An additional $75 billion was allocated to hospitals and other health care providers faced with COVID-19 revenue losses and cost challenges. The Disaster Loans Program received $50 billion, and $25 billion was allocated for testing, including $825 million designated for community health centers and rural health clinics.

Prospect for Further COVID-19 Legislation

Cassling considered the prospect for further legislative response to COVID-19 (as of June 25, 2020). Conflicting priorities between Republicans and Democrats make it difficult to predict what will happen next, she said. She also noted discussions of incentives to encourage a safe economic reopening versus a continued reliance on federal stimulus. Cassling said that support for rural hospitals comes up repeatedly in legislative discussions, reflecting substantial concern about the financial state of a number of hospitals, especially as COVID-19 cases rise in rural communities. In May 2020, Democrats passed a $3 trillion relief package through the House of Representatives that included every democratic priority related to the pandemic. However, the bill did not have enough support to pass through the Senate. She said that Democratic priorities for the next COVID-19 bill include funding for state and local governments, with an additional Federal Medical Assistance Percentages rate increase; further relief for health care providers, including rural hospitals; national plans for testing, contact tracing, and future vaccine distribution;

improving access to health insurance coverage;[17] addressing racial and ethnic health disparities; and support for essential workers, including health care providers, with a provision for hazard pay. Cassling concluded that in response to current unrest in the United States around issues of race, racial and ethnic health disparities have moved to the forefront of these priorities. Although bipartisan conversations are necessary for additional legislation to become law, this had yet to happen as of June 2020, she added.

DISCUSSION

Addressing Social Determinants of Health in Rural Settings

Noting that urban hospitals have access to support from community agencies, Murphy asked Putnam how SDOH are to be addressed in rural areas that lack this type of support. Putnam agreed that lack of access to community agencies is a challenge for rural providers, so ingenuity is required to address SDOH. He gave an example focused on behavioral health, mental health, and addiction needs. While rural providers are able to perform surgeries and treat conditions such as pneumonia, they do not have access to the range of services found in urban areas. Rural providers found that some patients were unable to manage their chronic diseases properly because of mental health issues, so they had to create their own programs. Putnam gave the perspective that mental health services are not "acute care," which fueled initial reluctance to expand these services. However, he suggested that over time, there has been increasing acknowledgment that rural providers should build programs to provide mental health services.

Putnam also emphasized the need to take advantage of available resources. In rural communities, social services are often not provided through formal programs, but instead come from area churches and other civic organizations. In the absence of government solutions, tightknit communities work together to address issues related to transportation needs and other barriers. Putnam gave an example of the lack of PPE as the pandemic began, saying that health care team members were becoming ill from exposure to COVID-19 because they were running out of masks. The community began sewing masks to build up the mask supply and protect the team. Community members have also volunteered to take

---

[17] Cassling noted that the Health and Economic Recovery Omnibus Emergency Solutions Act created a new special enrollment period for the Patient Protection and Affordable Care Act, as well as Consolidated Omnibus Budget Reconciliation Act coverage for people who had lost their jobs.

patients to physician appointments or to the pharmacy to have prescriptions filled. Creativity and community are required to address these barriers in the absence of formal programs, he emphasized, and he said that there is no single answer to the question of how to address SDOH without agency support. Instead, he said, there are "as many answers as there are small communities."

Rural Issues as National Issues

Murphy asked Mueller to comment on the view that challenges of rural communities are rural issues rather than national issues. She also asked how advocacy efforts can most effectively make this an issue of national prominence. Mueller replied that the interconnectedness of society allows us to see that we have much to learn from one another, and the pandemic has highlighted this. Rather than developing a demonstration in a city and scaling it down to rural, or scaling a rural demonstration up to urban, Mueller suggested examining the elements of each organization's or community's efforts and learning from those. He cited the House Committee on Ways and Means's newly formed Rural and Underserved Communities Health Task Force as an initiative that can determine relevant characteristics common at the neighborhood or community level. Mueller said the interconnectivity across urban and rural settings is already evident, but the new knowledge and innovations would be fostered more rapidly if the current siloed circumstances can be changed to allow more mutual learning from demonstrations.

Global Budgeting Model for Financial Stability

Murphy asked Mueller to comment further on the Pennsylvania Rural Health Initiative and global budgets. Mueller referenced a recent opinion piece from a group at Harvard University working on the Pennsylvania model (Fried et al., 2020). It made the case for global budgeting, as innovation often arises during a crisis but will be more effective with long-term stability in financing. As the global budgeting model provides annual budgets rather than dependence on billable services, this model would be more secure and flexible during crises such as a pandemic and its consequent lost revenue sources, he added.

Federal Response to the COVID-19 Navajo Nation Outbreak

Murphy asked Smith to provide his perspective on the federal response to the COVID-19 outbreak among the Navajo Nation, the challenges involved, and the steps that are being taken or that should be taken to prepare the entire population for the second wave of the virus. Smith responded that some tribes have been hit hard by COVID-19 more quickly than others, and tribal leaders and Indian urban organization leaders are discussing the best ways to prepare. Smith said that as COVID-19 continues to spread to other parts of the country, disseminating informational materials to tribal governments is key. IHS is relying heavily on CDC as the primary source of information, he noted. However, to ensure that the requisite tribal consultation and conferring with urban Indian organizations are taking place, IHS is taking an all-of-government approach. For instance, weekly calls with the White House Office of Intergovernmental Affairs have recently increased to biweekly frequency to create opportunities to hear the issues and needs firsthand. Smith stated that these communication chains have provided the most substantial and direct assistance in reaching directly to the top levels of government.

A unified coordination group is necessary, Smith said. This is occurring in the Navajo Nation, where the Navajo Nation partners with the federal government in a unified command to address the issues. Smith noted that challenges requiring amplified messaging range from access to PPE to broader issues—related to housing, for example—that are common in rural communities and perhaps even more frequent in Indian communities. He added that when multiple family members reside together in a small residence, it is difficult to maintain the proper social distance. Communication has been the cornerstone of IHS's approach to the COVID-19 pandemic thus far, said Smith. From helping with direct resources from the federal government to assisting with donations coming from philanthropies and churches, the pandemic response requires an all-of-government partnership approach.

Pandemic Response in Rural Areas

Putnam was asked to comment on the rural response to the COVID-19 pandemic. He responded that the limited number of ER physicians, respiratory therapists, and imaging technicians is a particular challenge for rural areas during a pandemic. When rural health professionals contract the virus and can no longer work because of illness and the potential to spread the virus to others, there are no other departments to pull workforce from. Therefore, Putnam advised rural facilities to plan for situations that can occur if rural health professionals test positive for COVID-19, such as closed ERs. He added that "there are no competitors during a pandemic" in describing the importance of collaborating in preparation efforts among hospitals, physicians' offices, dentists' offices, and nursing homes.

As rural facilities have communicated their needs, communication and resources have been shared across state lines, said Putnam. He said his top priority has been protecting his team, but he has faced severe shortages in PPE such as N95s, controlled air purifying respirators, powered air purifying respirators, regular masks, and isolation gowns. It has been a difficult leadership challenge to keep his team safe in the absence of adequate protective equipment, he emphasized. However, facilities have worked together to address the PPE shortages. For example, other hospitals have offered to share what little surplus of equipment they have, and dentist offices have offered to shut down for 1 week to make masks available for the hospital.

Rural Policy Initiatives

Murphy remarked that before the COVID-19 pandemic hit, she and other colleagues who are focused on rural health policy felt momentum building for this policy area. She asked Cassling what rural policies to expect moving forward and whether she feels that rural policy has a strong foothold in national politics. Cassling stated that there will be many opportunities for action on rural health priorities. The most evident is the telehealth movement, which has strong bipartisan support for its continued expansion because of the benefits it has shown during the pandemic. She sees the expansion of telehealth as a long-standing outcome of the pandemic, but it will take time to address hospital infrastructure issues that may pose barriers to the expansion. Potential also exists for new models, Cassling said, noting Senator Chuck Grassley's work to establish a new rural hospital model with more flexibility for communities. In the House of Representatives, Congressman Jodey Arrington is leading the effort for a new model. Cassling said that bipartisan conversations in this area are taking place, but working out the details will be a lengthy process. Cassling concluded that addressing the COVID-19 pandemic has been the central focus of Congress, and whether or not another stimulus package or appropriations bill will be passed is uncertain. Similarly, it is unknown whether any efforts not directly related to addressing the pandemic or funding the government through the end of the year will be feasible.

Role of Electronic Health Records in Rural Care

Murphy asked Smith about policies or regulatory provisions that might be helpful in moving forward with EHRs in tribal communities. Smith replied that tribal health programs have explored commercial products in an effort to find their own solutions to sharing information with IHS. He noted that IHS received additional resources before the COVID-19 pandemic from HHS to examine various EHR platforms and that IHS has also worked with the Department of Veterans Affairs to learn from their process of EHR modernization. Tribes that cover multiple states are a particular challenge for EHRs, Smith noted. For example, the Navajo Nation covers parts of Arizona, New Mexico, and Utah. Smith said that the current telehealth expansion has presented new opportunities, and IHS is working with other federal agencies (e.g., the Federal Communications Commission) to enter into broadband expansion on tribal lands. Additionally, some COVID-19 funding supplements for information technology will enable continued efforts toward EHR modernization.

Murphy closed the final panel of the workshop by thanking the speakers, the National Academies staff, and the workshop planning committee members for organizing the virtual event.

Appendix A

Speaker and Planning Committee Member Biosketches[1]

Rhonda Barcus, M.S., L.P.C., joined the National Rural Health Resource Center in 2012 and manages the Small Rural Hospital Transition Project and population and community health services. She has worked in hospital settings since 1987. Ms. Barcus is experienced in leadership and organizational development and has assisted hospitals to address organization-wide goals related to improving patient experience and staff retention. Ms. Barcus received her M.S. in psychology from Georgia College & State University. She is also a licensed professional counselor and has worked in the field of substance use.

Darrold Bertsch is the chief executive officer (CEO) of the Sakakawea Medical Center, a critical access hospital located in Hazen, North Dakota, and is also the CEO of the Coal Country Community Health Center, a federally qualified health center with four service delivery sites in west central North Dakota. Mr. Bertsch has served in this unique shared CEO role for the past 9 years, leading collaborative efforts that have improved the delivery of patient care and the development of a patient-centered medical neighborhood of care. Mr. Bertsch has worked in health care for 46 years, with the last 26 as a CEO. Mr. Bertsch is an active proponent of rural health care and serves on various local, state, and national boards and committees.

---

[1] * Denotes planning committee member, † denotes roundtable member.

Michael E. Bird, M.S.W., M.P.H.,* is the public health program director for the Indian Health Council. Mr. Bird has more than 30 years of public health experience in the areas of medical social work, substance abuse prevention, health promotion and disease prevention, HIV/AIDS prevention, behavioral health, and health care administration. He is the first American Indian and social worker to serve as the president (2000–2001) of the American Public Health Association. He is also the past president of the New Mexico Public Health Association and was a fellow in the U.S. Public Health Service Primary Care Policy Fellowship Program. Mr. Bird has served on the boards of the Kewa Pueblo Health Corporation, American Indian Graduate Center, Bernalillo County Off Reservation Native American Commission, Health Action New Mexico, Seva Foundation, National Collaborating Centre for Aboriginal Health Advisory Committee (Canada), and AARP National Policy Council. He earned an M.S.W. from The University of Utah and an M.P.H. at the University of California (UC), Berkeley. In 2018 he was honored by the UC Berkeley School of Public Health as one of the most influential public health alumni in the institution's 75-year history.

Daniel Calac, M.D., has served as the chief medical officer of the Indian Health Council located near San Diego, California, since 2003. He was raised on the Pauma Indian Reservation and graduated from San Diego State University. Dr. Calac attended Harvard Medical School and completed his internship and residency at the University of Southern California–Los Angeles County Combined Internal Medicine/Pediatrics Residency Program. He is board certified in both internal medicine and pediatrics. He also practices hospice/palliative care medicine and is board eligible in this field. He is a member of the Pauma Band of Luiseno Indians and is actively involved in his community. His professional interests include chronic disease and clinical research. Dr. Calac serves as the principal investigator for the California Native American Research Center for Health, which is a project funded by the National Institutes of Health that provides a platform for community-based participatory research in American Indian communities. He is actively engaged in several research projects that aim to improve the health of American Indians and encourage students to pursue careers as scientists and/or health care professionals. Dr. Calac also serves on a variety of committees, including the Health Research Advisory Council for the Department of Health and Human Services, the Committee on Native American Child Health, the Cal State San Marcos Foundation Board, and the governance board for the All Tribes American Indian Charter School.

Tim Callaghan, Ph.D., M.A., has research interests in health politics, the Patient Protection and Affordable Care Act, autism policy, opioid policy, rural health policy, state politics, and public opinion about health topics. He is an assistant professor in the Department of Health Policy and Management at the Texas A&M University School of Public Health. Dr. Callaghan has had research featured in prominent journals, including the *American Journal of Public Health*; *Journal of Health Politics, Policy, and Law*; *American Politics Research*; *Social Science and Medicine*; and *Publius: The Journal of Federalism*. He serves on the advisory board of the Program in Health Law and Policy and is also the director of evaluation with the nationally recognized Southwest Rural Health Research Center at Texas A&M University. The center, funded by the Health Resources and Services Administration's Federal Office of Rural Health Policy, was established to address the needs of rural and underserved populations across Texas and the nation by bringing together a unique combination of faculty expertise in health policy, health economics, aging, long-term care, health law, epidemiology, biostatistics, and chronic disease. Dr. Callaghan received his B.A. in political science and B.S. in biological sciences from the University of Connecticut. He then went on to receive his M.A. and Ph.D. in political science from the University of Minnesota, Twin Cities.

Kate Cassling, M.A., is a director with the Bipartisan Policy Center (BPC) Action where she works on health care policy advocacy. Prior to joining BPC Action, Ms. Cassling worked for more than 8 years on Capitol Hill, most recently serving as a legislative assistant for Senator Joe Manchin, specializing in health care, education, and labor policy. In that role, she managed the senator's work on the Senate Appropriations Labor, Health and Human Services, Education, and Related Agencies Subcommittee and the Joint Select Committee on Solvency of Multiemployer Pension Plans. Previously, she worked as a legislative assistant to Congresswoman Dina Titus and as a legislative aide to Senator Susan Collins. Ms. Cassling has a B.A. in economics from Swarthmore College and an M.A. in education from Tel Aviv University.

Jan Marie Eberth, Ph.D., M.S.P.H., is an associate professor of epidemiology and the director of the Rural and Minority Health Research Center at the University of South Carolina. Dr. Eberth conducts research in the areas of health geography, social epidemiology, and cancer prevention and control. As the director of the Rural and Minority Health Research Center at the Arnold School of Public Health, Dr. Eberth works with investigators across the university to identify and address problems experienced by rural and minority populations in order to guide research, policy, and related advocacy. She received her M.S.P.H. in epidemiology from the

Texas A&M Health Science Center in the School of Rural Public Health in 2006 and her Ph.D. in epidemiology from the University of Texas Health Science Center in the School of Public Health in 2011. Dr. Eberth also completed a National Cancer Institute–funded postdoctoral fellowship at the University of Texas MD Anderson Cancer Center in 2012.

Alva Ferdinand, Dr.P.H., J.D.,[*] is an assistant professor in the Department of Health Policy and Management at the Texas A&M School of Public Health. She also serves as the director of the Southwest Rural Health Research Center at the School of Public Health. Her research interests are health laws and ethics, disparities in health outcomes, research integrity, state and federal regulation in health care delivery, and effectiveness of laws aimed at improving public health. Dr. Ferdinand has examined such issues as the effect of tax-exemption status on the provision of community benefits among various hospital ownership types, the relationship between neighborhood built environments and physical activity, the effect of strict immigration laws on health services utilization among immigrant populations, and the effects of texting-while-driving bans on roadway safety. She has also examined issues of mental health, access to care, and diabetes in rural areas. Dr. Ferdinand has been called on to provide expert testimony to state and federal legislative bodies on the effectiveness of laws aimed at improving public health. She holds a J.D. from the Michigan State University College of Law and a Dr.P.H. from The University of Alabama at Birmingham.

Katharine Ferguson, M.P.A., is the associate director of The Aspen Institute Community Strategies Group (CSG) and the director of CSG's Rural and Regional Initiatives. Before joining The Aspen Institute, Ms. Ferguson served in the Obama administration as the chief of staff for the White House Domestic Policy Council and as the chief of staff for rural development at the U.S. Department of Agriculture. Previously, Ms. Ferguson worked on the Senate Committee on Agriculture and as staff to multiple U.S. senators on topics ranging from community economic development and economic mobility to conservation, agriculture, food, public health, and nutrition. Committed to bridging perceived divides and advancing equity, regardless of the topic at hand, Ms. Ferguson is interested in the practical challenges of civic engagement, institution building, systems change, and governance. In 2018, she served on the transition team for Colorado Attorney General Phil Weiser. She currently serves on the Steering Committee for the Western Governors' Association's Reimagining the Rural West Initiative, and the Service Year Alliance Rural Policy Advisory Council, and she was recently appointed to Colorado's Just Transition Advisory Committee. A graduate of Tufts University, Ms. Ferguson holds an M.P.A. from the Maxwell School of Citizenship and Public Affairs at Syracuse University.

Mark Holmes, Ph.D., is a professor in the Department of Health Policy and Management in the University of North Carolina Gillings School of Global Public Health, the director of the North Carolina Rural Health Research and Policy Analysis Center, and the director of the Cecil G. Sheps Center for Health Services Research, where he is also the co-director of the Program on Health Care Economics and Finance. His interests include hospital finance, rural health, workforce, health policy, and patient-centered outcomes research. In 2014, Dr. Holmes received the Phillip and Ruth Hettleman Prize for Artistic and Scholarly Achievement by Young Faculty. In 2015 he was named Outstanding Researcher by the National Rural Health Association. Previously, he was the vice president of the North Carolina Institute of Medicine, where he gained experience in North Carolina health policy. He previously served on the board of the North Carolina Health Insurance Risk Pool. His state policy work led to his 2010 Health Care Hero "Rising Star" award from the *Triangle Business Journal*. He is a member of the editorial boards of the *Journal of Rural Health* and the *North Carolina Medical Journal*. He received his B.S. in mathematics and economics from Michigan State University and his Ph.D. from the Department of Economics at the University of North Carolina at Chapel Hill.

Alana Knudson, Ph.D., M.Ed.,* is a principal research scientist and the co-director of the Walsh Center for Rural Health Analysis at NORC at the University of Chicago. Dr. Knudson is also the deputy director for the Rural Health Reform Policy Research Center, one of seven rural health research centers funded by the Federal Office of Rural Health Policy. She has 20 years of experience implementing and directing public health programs, leading health services and health policy research projects, and evaluating the effects of programs. She conducted numerous health services research studies, health policy studies, and public health projects funded by the Agency for Healthcare Research and Quality, Centers for Disease Control and Prevention, Centers for Medicare & Medicaid Services, Center for Medicare & Medicaid Innovation, Health Resources and Services Administration, Administration for Children and Families, U.S. Agency for International Development, and Robert Wood Johnson Foundation. Her research and policy project findings have informed state, tribal, and federal health policy. She also has state and national public health experience, having worked at the North Dakota Department of Health and for the Association of State and Territorial Health Officials.

Dr. Knudson earned a dual master of education degree and a Ph.D. from Oregon State University in Corvallis, Oregon.

Sanne Magnan, M.D., Ph.D.,† is the co-chair of the Roundtable on Population Health Improvement of the National Academies of Sciences, Engineering, and Medicine. She is the former president (2006–2007) and the chief executive officer (2011–2016) of the Institute for Clinical Systems Improvement. In 2007, she was appointed the commissioner of the Minnesota Department of Health by Minnesota Governor Tim Pawlenty. She served from 2007 to 2010 and had significant responsibility for the implementation of Minnesota's 2008 health reform legislation, including the Statewide Health Improvement Program, standardized quality reporting, development of provider peer grouping, certification process for health care homes, and baskets of care. Dr. Magnan was a staff physician at the Tuberculosis Clinic at the St. Paul–Ramsey County Department of Public Health (2002–2015). She was a member of the Population-based Payment Model Workgroup of the Healthcare Payment Learning and Action Network (2015–2016) and a member of the Centers for Medicare & Medicaid Services Multisector Collaboration Measure Development Technical Expert Panel (2016). She is on Epic's Population Health Steering Board and on the Healthy People 2030 Engagement Subcommittee. She served on the board of MN Community Measurement and the board of NorthPoint Health & Wellness Center, a federally qualified health center and part of Hennepin Health. Her previous experience also includes the vice president and the medical director of Consumer Health at Blue Cross and Blue Shield of Minnesota. Currently, she is a senior fellow with HealthPartners Institute and an adjunct assistant professor of medicine at the University of Minnesota. Dr. Magnan holds an M.D. and a Ph.D. in medicinal chemistry from the University of Minnesota and is a board-certified internist.

Nir Menachemi, Ph.D., M.P.H., is the Fairbanks Endowed Chair and serves as the chair of the Health Policy and Management Department of the Indiana University Richard M. Fairbanks School of Public Health. He holds the rank of professor. Dr. Menachemi also holds an appointment as a scientist with the Regenstrief Institute, an internationally recognized informatics and health care research organization that is dedicated to the improvement of health through research that enhances the quality and cost-effectiveness of health care. Before joining the Fairbanks School of Public Health, Dr. Menachemi held faculty positions at The University of Alabama at Birmingham School of Public Health and the Florida State University College of Medicine. He has published more than 200 peer-reviewed scientific papers, and his work has appeared in numerous prestigious professional journals, including the *New England Journal of Medicine*, *Health Affairs*, *Health Services Research*, and the *American Journal of Public Health*. Dr. Menachemi's research examines how organizational strategies (e.g., health information technology adoption) affect critical performance measures, including quality outcomes and financial performance. In addition, he has published extensively on health policy and public health topics ranging from obesity issues to the effects of various laws or policies on health outcomes. Dr. Menachemi's work has been funded by such diverse entities as the Centers for Disease Control and Prevention, the Centers for Medicare & Medicaid Services, and private foundations and corporations. In addition, Dr. Menachemi has developed several long-term partnerships with health departments at the state and local level in both Alabama and Florida. More recently, he has begun similar partnerships with state and local entities in Indiana.

Karen Minyard, Ph.D., M.N., has been the director of the Georgia Health Policy Center (GHPC) since 2001 and is also a research professor with the Georgia State University Department of Public Management and Policy. Dr. Minyard connects the research, policy, and programmatic work of the center across issue areas including population health, health philanthropy, public and private health coverage, and the uninsured. Dr. Minyard has experience with the state Medicaid program, with both the design of program reforms and external evaluation. Her research interests include financing and evaluation of health-related social policy programs; strategic alignment of public and private health policy through collective impact; the role of local health initiatives in access and health improvement; the role of targeted technical assistance in improving the sustainability, efficiency, and programmatic effectiveness of nonprofit health collaboratives; and health and health care financing. In addition to overseeing the center's overall strategic vision, Dr. Minyard plays a leadership role in several center projects that weave together the key learnings, skill sets, and areas of expertise of GHPC, including evaluation, technical assistance, policy and economic analysis, backbone and organizational support, health and health care financing, health system transformation, Health in All Policies, and rural health. She is currently the co-principal investigator and is spearheading evaluation efforts for GHPC's national coordinating center, Bridging for Health: Improving Community Health Through Innovations in Financing, sponsored by the Robert Wood Johnson Foundation. She also serves on the executive trio of the Atlanta Regional Collaborative for Health Improvement, along with the Atlanta Regional Commission and the United Way of Greater Atlanta.

José T. Montero, M.D., M.H.C.D.S.,*† is the director of the Centers for Disease Control and Prevention's (CDC's) Center for State, Tribal, Local, and Territorial Support, where he oversees support to the U.S. health departments and those serving tribal nations and insular areas. He provides leadership for key activities and technical assistance designed to improve the public health system's capacity and performance to achieve the nation's goals in population health. With his team, Dr. Montero leads efforts to create communities of practice where CDC's senior leaders work with the executive leaders of the public health jurisdictions, key partners, and stakeholders to identify new, improved, or innovative strategies to prepare the public health system to respond to changing environments. Previously, Dr. Montero served as the vice president of population health and health system integration at Cheshire Medical Center/Dartmouth-Hitchcock Keene. He has also served as the director of the Division of Public Health Services at the New Hampshire Department of Health and Human Services. Dr. Montero has held many national and regional committee leadership positions, including serving as the president of the board of directors of the Association of State and Territorial Health Officials (ASTHO) and the chair of ASTHO's Infectious Diseases Policy Committee. Dr. Montero has an M.D. from the Universidad Nacional de Colombia. He specialized in family medicine and completed his residency at the Universidad del Valle in Cali, Colombia. He also holds an epidemiology degree from Pontificia Universidad Javeriana in Bogotá, Colombia, and he received his certification of field epidemiology from the Colombia Field Epidemiology Training Program and an M.H.C.D.S. from Dartmouth College.

Paul Moore, Ph.D., is a senior health policy advisor to the Federal Office of Rural Health Policy, which is part of the Health Resources and Services Administration. Dr. Moore has a lifetime of experience related to rural health care, including more than 30 years in community and hospital pharmacy. He has also served as the chief executive officer of a county health care authority, consisting of one of the nation's earliest critical access hospitals, the county emergency medical services, a physician clinic, and a home health agency. Dr. Moore is also a past president of the National Rural Health Association and currently serves as the executive secretary for the National Advisory Committee for Rural Health and Human Services.

Tom Morris, M.P.A.,* serves as the associate administrator for rural health policy in the Health Resources and Services Administration (HRSA) of the Department of Health and Human Services (HHS). In that role, Mr. Morris oversees the work of the Federal Office of Rural Health Policy, which is charged with advising the Secretary of HHS on rural health issues. In 2012, he was the recipient of the HHS Distinguished Service Award, and in 2015 he was awarded a Presidential Rank Award for Meritorious Service. Over the course of his federal career, Mr. Morris has testified on rural health issues before the House and Senate. He has past work experience in the Senate as well as various policy and program positions within HRSA and HHS. A 1996 Presidential Management Intern, Mr. Morris came to government after a career as a newspaper reporter and editor. He has an undergraduate degree in journalism from the University of North Carolina at Chapel Hill and an M.P.A. with a concentration in community health from East Carolina University. He also earned a certificate in public leadership from the Brookings Institution in 2008.

Keith J. Mueller, Ph.D., M.A., is the Gerhard Hartman Professor and the head of the Department of Health Management and Policy at The University of Iowa. He is also the director of the Rural Policy Research Institute (RUPRI) Center for Rural Health Policy Analysis and the chair of the RUPRI Health Panel. He has served as the president of the National Rural Health Association (NRHA) and as a member of the National Advisory Committee on Rural Health and Human Services. He has also served on national advisory committees to the Agency for Healthcare Research and Quality and the Centers for Medicare & Medicaid Services. He has published more than 220 scholarly articles and policy papers and received awards recognizing his research contributions from NRHA, RUPRI, and the University of Nebraska. In 2016, he received The University of Iowa Regents Award for Faculty Excellence. His Ph.D. is in political science from the University of Arizona, and he completed a faculty fellowship with Johns Hopkins University.

Karen Murphy, Ph.D., M.B.A., R.N.,*† is the executive vice president, the chief innovation officer, and the founding director of The Steele Institute for Health Innovation at Geisinger. Dr. Murphy has worked to improve and transform health care delivery throughout her career in both the public and private sectors. Before joining Geisinger, she served as Pennsylvania's secretary of health, addressing the most significant health issues facing the state, including the opioid epidemic. Prior to her role as secretary, Dr. Murphy served as the director of the State Innovation Models Initiative at the Centers for Medicare & Medicaid Services (CMS), leading a $990 million CMS investment designed to accelerate health care innovation across the United States. She previously served as the president and the chief executive officer (CEO) of the Moses Taylor Health Care System in Scranton, Pennsylvania, and as the founder and the CEO of Physicians Health Alliance, Inc., an integrated medical group practice within Moses Taylor. Dr. Murphy earned her Ph.D. in business administration from the Temple University Fox School of Business. She holds an M.B.A. from Marywood University, a B.S. in liberal arts from the University of Scranton, and a diploma in nursing from the Scranton State Hospital School of Nursing.

Valerie Nurr'araaluk Davidson, a Yup'ik and enrolled tribal member of the Orutsaramiut Traditional Native Council of Bethel, serves as the first female president of Alaska Pacific University. Ms. Nurr'araaluk Davidson's prior 20-year health career included state service as the commissioner of the Alaska Department of Health & Social Services, where she implemented Medicaid Expansion, Medicaid Reform, and the Alaska Tribal Child Welfare Compact. Ms. Nurr'araaluk Davidson later served as Alaska's first Alaska Native female lieutenant governor in the final weeks of the Walker administration. Ms. Nurr'araaluk Davidson began her tribal health career at the Yukon Kuskokwim Health Corporation and the Alaska Native Tribal Health Consortium.

Lars Peterson, Ph.D., M.D.,* is a family physician and a health services researcher who serves as the vice president of research for the American Board of Family Medicine (ABFM). He also has an appointment as an associate professor of family and community medicine in the University of Kentucky's Rural & Underserved Health Research Center, where he provides direct clinical care and teaches students and residents. Dr. Peterson, a native of Utah, received his medical and graduate degrees from Case Western Reserve University in Cleveland, Ohio, and completed his family medicine residency at the Trident/Medical University of South Carolina family medicine residency program. At ABFM, Dr. Peterson leads a research team focused on elucidating the outcomes of family medicine certification, particularly the effects that certification activities have on the quality of care delivered by family physicians. In addition, Dr. Peterson and his team seek to understand the ecology of family medicine over time—what physicians do in practice and their contribution to high-quality health care. His research interests also include investigating associations between area-level measures of health care and socioeconomics with both health and access to health care, rural health, primary care, and comprehensiveness of primary care. Dr. Peterson has authored more than 100 peer-reviewed publications and made more than 100 national and international conference presentations.

Janice C. Probst, Ph.D., M.S., is a distinguished professor emerita at the University of South Carolina Arnold School of Public Health. Dr. Probst is a nationally recognized researcher in the areas of health services and policy, with a specific focus on rural health and health disparities. She was a founding faculty member for the Rural and Minority Health Research Center (formerly, the South Carolina Rural Health Research Center), which was established in 2000. She has more than 140 peer-reviewed scientific publications, along with more than 200 presentations at scientific conferences. Dr. Probst is a member of the National Rural Health Association Health Equity Council and serves on the board of directors of the South Carolina Office of Rural Health. Dr. Probst completed her B.A. at Duke University, her M.S. at Purdue University, and her Ph.D. at the University of South Carolina.

Tim Putnam, D.H.A., M.B.A., F.A.C.H.E., is the president and the chief executive officer of Margaret Mary Health in Batesville, Indiana, and has more than 30 years of health care experience. He received his D.H.A. from the Medical University of South Carolina, where his dissertation was focused on acute stroke care in rural hospitals. He currently chairs the National Rural Health Association's Policy Congress, the National Rural Accountable Care Consortium, and was appointed by the governor to the Indiana Board of Graduate Medical Education, which he also chairs. In 2015, Dr. Putnam was certified as an Emergency Medical Technician and serves on the Batesville Fire and EMS Lifesquad.

Allen Smart, M.P.H., M.A., is a national spokesperson and an advocate for improving rural philanthropic practice under his group PhilanthropywoRx. In addition, he recently completed a role as the project director for a national rural philanthropic project partially supported by the Robert Wood Johnson Foundation and based at Campbell University in Buies Creek, North Carolina. He regularly consults with regional and national foundations on rural and philanthropic strategy. Mr. Smart is the former interim president, the vice president of programs, and the director of the Health Care Division at the Kate B. Reynolds Charitable Trust. Prior to coming to the Trust in 2006, Mr. Smart was the vice president of programs at the Rapides Foundation, a health care conversion funder in Alexandria, Louisiana. He has also served as the director of community development for a midwestern Catholic Hospital System and as the grants administrator for the City of Santa Monica, California. Mr. Smart received his M.P.H. from the University of Illinois at Chicago, his M.A. in telecommunication arts from the University of Michigan, and his B.A. in philosophy from Macalester College. As part of his personal and professional interest in philanthropy, Mr. Smart regularly writes for sites such as *The Daily Yonder*, *Inside Philanthropy*, and *Grantcraft and Exponent Philanthropy* and presents to national and regional organizations like Grantmakers in Health, the Southeastern Council of Foundations, the National Rural Assembly, and the Federal Office of Rural Health Policy. He is a member of the National Advisory Committee for the Rural Resource Hub at the University of North Dakota; the Culture of Health Prize Selection Committee for the Robert Wood Johnson Foundation; the board of directors for Healthy Communities by Design; and the board of the North Carolina Healthcare Association Foundation.

P. Benjamin Smith, M.B.A., M.A., is an enrolled member of the Navajo Nation and the deputy director for intergovernmental affairs for the Indian Health Service (IHS). IHS, an agency within the Department of Health and Human Services, is the principal federal health care provider and health advocate for American Indians and Alaska Natives. As the deputy director for intergovernmental affairs, Mr. Smith provides leadership on tribal and urban Indian health activities, particulary the implementation of the Title I and Title V authorities under the Indian Self-Determination and Education Assistance Act and Title V of the Indian Health Care Improvement Act, through oversight of the Office of Tribal Self-Governance, the Office of Direct Service and Contracting Tribes, and the Office of Urban Indian Health Programs. Mr. Smith previously served as the director of the Office of Tribal Self-Governance, where he oversaw all aspects of the administration of the Tribal Self-Governance Program, authorized by Title V of the Indian Self-Determination and Education Assistance Act. Prior to his federal service, Mr. Smith worked as a self-governance specialist for the Choctaw Nation of Oklahoma, performing research, advisory services, and consultation on health programs with national, state, and local health departments. Throughout his career, Mr. Smith has received numerous awards, including the 2014 Arthur S. Flemming Award from The George Washington University Trachtenberg School of Public Policy and Public Administration, which honors outstanding federal employees for their exceptional contributions to the federal government. He has also received several IHS National Director's Awards for his contributions to tribal consultation activities, IHS Strategic Plan updates, and the agency lead negotiators curriculum. Mr. Smith received his M.B.A. from The George Washington University, an M.A. in international peace and conflict resolution from American University, and a B.A. from Brigham Young University. He is also one of the Navajo Nation's Chief Manuelito Scholars.

Sirin Yaemsiri, Ph.D., M.S.P.H., is a senior statistician at the U.S. Government Accountability Office. Previously, she was a health statistician at the National Center for Health Statistics at the Centers for Disease Control and Prevention, where she provided data expertise to the Healthy People 2020 initiative. In addition to rural health, Dr. Yaemsiri's areas of interest include vital statistics, health disparities, developing key indicators, assessing data quality, statistics, and data visualization. Dr. Yaemsiri holds a Ph.D. in epidemiology from the University of North Carolina at Chapel Hill and is an adjunct professor at the University of Maryland, College Park.

Appendix B

Workshop Agenda

Population Health in Rural America in 2020

June 24–25, 2020

Wednesday, June 24

11 AM	**Welcome**	**Sanne Magnan,** Roundtable Co-Chair, HealthPartners Institute
	Rural America in Context	Rural Demographics and Social Determinants of Health **Alana Knudson,** Walsh Center for Rural Health Analysis, NORC at the University of Chicago Structural Urbanism: Current Funding Mechanisms Systematically Disadvantage Rural Populations **Janice Probst,** Arnold School of Public Health, University of South Carolina Moderator: **Lars Peterson,** Rural & Underserved Health Research Center, University of Kentucky

	Rural Health Vital Signs	Why Is Mortality Higher in Rural Areas? **Mark Holmes,** North Carolina Rural Health Research and Policy Analysis Center, University of North Carolina at Chapel Hill
		Tribal Public Health Activities **Valerie Nurr'araaluk Davidson,** Alaska Pacific University
		Rural Data Challenges in Healthy People 2020 **Sirin Yaemsiri,** U.S. Government Accountability Office
		Looking Ahead: Rural Healthy People 2030 Process and Rural Health Indicators **Alva Ferdinand,** Southwest Rural Health Research Center, Texas A&M University
		Do Rural Racial Disparities Get Lost in the Larger Discussion on Rural and Urban Disparities? **Jan Eberth,** Rural and Minority Health Research Center, University of South Carolina
		Moderator: **Alana Knudson,** Walsh Center for Rural Health Analysis, NORC at the University of Chicago
1 PM		**Lunch Break**
2 PM	**Health Care in Action**	Rural Health Care Landscape **Paul Moore,** Federal Office of Rural Health Policy, Health Resources and Services Administration
		Tribal Health Care in Rural Settings **Daniel Calac,** Indian Health Council
		Wraparound Services: Implications for Rural America **Nir Menachemi,** Indiana University–Purdue University Indianapolis

APPENDIX B   133

| | | The Role of Community Health Workers in Addressing the Needs of Rural Americans
Timothy Callaghan, Southwest Rural Health Research Center, Texas A&M University |

Moderator: **Tom Morris,** Federal Office of Rural Health Policy, Health Resources and Services Administration

Thursday, June 25

| 11 AM | **Welcome Day 2** | **Joshua Sharfstein,** Roundtable Co-Chair, Johns Hopkins Bloomberg School of Public Health |
| | **Assessment and Implementation Strategies for Rural Population Health Improvement** | Coordinated Community Health Needs Assessments and Population Health
Darrold Bertsch, Sakakawea Medical Center and Coal Country Community Health Center |

Supporting Population Health Efforts: Minnesota Integrated Behavioral Program
Rhonda Barcus, National Rural Health Research Center

Connecting Rural Development, Health, and Opportunity: The Role of Rural Development Hubs and Policy
Katharine Ferguson, The Aspen Institute Community Strategies Group

Innovations in Sustaining Rural Population Health
Karen Minyard, Georgia Health Policy Center

Moderator: **Allen Smart,** PhilanthropywoRx

| 1 PM | | **Lunch Break** |

2 PM	**Rural Health Policy**	Rural Health Policy and Practice Toward Value-Based Care **Tim Putnam,** Mary Margaret Health, Indiana
		Confronting Rural America's Health Care Crisis: Bipartisan Policy Center Rural Health Task Force Recommendations **Keith Mueller,** Rural Policy Research Institute, College of Public Health, The University of Iowa
		Tribal Rural Health Policy **Benjamin Smith,** Indian Health Service
		The CARES Act **Kate Cassling,** Bipartisan Policy Center Action
		Moderator: **Karen Murphy,** The Steele Institute for Health Innovation, Geisinger
3:30 PM	**Closing Remarks**	Karen Murphy

Appendix C

References

AHRQ (Agency for Healthcare Research and Quality). 2017. *National healthcare quality and disparities report chartbook on rural health care.* AHRQ Pub. No. 17(18)-0001-2-EF.
The Aspen Institute Community Strategies Group. 2019. *Rural development hubs: Strengthening America's rural innovation infrastructure.* Washington, DC: The Aspen Institute.
Bolin, J. N., G. Bellamy, A. O. Ferdinand, B. A. Kash, and J. W. Helduser. 2015. *Rural healthy people 2020.* Volumes I and II. College Station, TX: Texas A&M Health Science Center School of Public Health, Southwest Rural Health Research Center.
Bond Edmond, M., L. Aletraris, and P. M. Roman. 2015. Rural substance use treatment centers in the United States: An assessment of treatment quality by location. *American Journal of Drug and Alcohol Abuse* 41(5):449–457.
Caldwell, J. T., C. L. Ford, S. P. Wallace, M. C. Wang, and L. M. Takahashi. 2016. Intersection of living in a rural versus urban area and race/ethnicity in explaining access to health care in the United States. *American Journal of Public Health* 106(8):1463–1469.
Callaghan, T., D. J. Washburn, K. Nimmons, D. Duchicela, A. Gurram, and J. Burdine. 2019. Immigrant health access in Texas: Policy, rhetoric, and fear in the Trump era. *BMC Health Services Research* 19(1):342.
Cromartie, J. 2018. *Rural America at a glance, 2018 edition.* Washington, DC: Economic Research Service, U.S. Department of Agriculture.
Ferguson, K., T. Pipa, and N. Geismar. 2020. *Redesign required: Principles for reimagining federal rural policy in the COVID-19 era.* Washington, DC: The Aspen Institute.
Fried, J. E., D. T. Liebers, and E. T. Roberts. 2020. Sustaining rural hospitals after COVID-19: The case for global budgets. *JAMA* 324(2):137–138.
Frieden, T. R. 2010. A framework for public health action: The health impact pyramid. *American Journal of Public Health* 100(4):590–595.
Gamm, L., L. Hutchison, B. Dabney, and A. Dorsey. 2010. *Rural Healthy People 2010: A companion document to Healthy People 2010.* College Station, TX: Texas A&M University System Health Science Center, School of Rural Public Health Southwest Rural Health Research Center.

Gonsalves, G. S., and F. W. Crawford. 2018. Dynamics of the HIV outbreak and response in Scott County, IN, USA, 2011–2015: A modelling study. *Lancet HIV* 5(10):e569–e577.

Goodnough, A. 2020. A tiny hospital struggles to treat a burst of coronavirus patients. *The New York Times*. https://www.nytimes.com/2020/04/16/health/coronavirus-rural-hospitals.html (accessed January 5, 2021).

Gottlieb, L. M., D. Hessler, D. Long, E. Laves, A. R. Burns, A. Amaya, P. Sweeney, C. Schudel, and N. E. Adler. 2016. Effects of social needs screening and in-person service navigation on child health: A randomized clinical trial. *JAMA Pediatrics* 170(11):e162521.

Hennessy, T. W., T. Ritter, R. C. Holman, D. L. Bruden, K. L. Yorita, L. Bulkow, J. E. Cheek, R. J. Singleton, and J. Smith. 2008. The relationship between in-home water service and the risk of respiratory tract, skin, and gastrointestinal tract infections among rural Alaska natives. *American Journal of Public Health* 98(11):2072–2078.

Holmes, M., and K. Thompson. 2019. *Risk factors and potentially preventable deaths in rural communities*. Chapel Hill, NC: North Carolina Rural Health Research Program.

James, B. C., and G. P. Poulsen. 2016. The case for capitation. *Harvard Business Review* 94(7–8):102–111.

James, C. V., R. Moonesinghe, S. M. Wilson-Frederick, J. E. Hall, A. Penman-Aguilar, and K. Bouye. 2017. Racial/ethnic health disparities among rural adults—United States, 2012–2015. *Morbidity and Mortality Weekly Report Surveillance Summary* 66(23):1–9.

June-Ho Kim, E. D., and M. B. Cole. 2020. How the rapid shift to telehealth leaves many community health centers behind during the COVID-19 pandemic. *Health Affairs Blog*. https://www.healthaffairs.org/do/10.1377/hblog20200529.449762/full (accessed January 5, 2021).

Khan, S. Q., A. Berrington de Gonzalez, A. F. Best, Y. Chen, E. A. Haozous, E. J. Rodriquez, S. Spillane, D. A. Thomas, D. Withrow, N. D. Freedman, and M. S. Shiels. 2018. Infant and youth mortality trends by race/ethnicity and cause of death in the United States. *JAMA Pediatrics* 172(12):e183317.

Larson, J. E., J. P. Leider, and A. Knudson. 2019. A practice report from the Northern Dental Access Center offering wraparound services at a community dental access clinic to improve treatment outcomes among rural populations in poverty. *Journal of Public Health Management and Practice* 25(5).

Lorch, S. A., and E. Enlow. 2016. The role of social determinants in explaining racial/ethnic disparities in perinatal outcomes. *Pediatric Research* 79(1–2):141–147.

MedPAC (Medicare Payment Advisory Commission). 2017. *Report to the Congress: Medicare payment policy*. P. 248.

Millett, G. A., A. T. Jones, D. Benkeser, S. Baral, L. Mercer, C. Beyrer, B. Honermann, E. Lankiewicz, L. Mena, J. S. Crowley, J. Sherwood, and P. S. Sullivan. 2020. Assessing differential impacts of COVID-19 on Black communities. *Annals of Epidemiology* 47:37–44.

Mitchell, L. J., L. E. Ball, L. J. Ross, K. A. Barnes, and L. T. Williams. 2017. Effectiveness of dietetic consultations in primary health care: A systematic review of randomized controlled trials. *Journal of the Academy of Nutrition and Dietetics* 117(12):1941–1962.

Mueller, K. J., A. F. Coburn, A. Knudson, J. P. Lundblad, A. C. MacKinney, and T. D. McBride. 2020. *Considerations for defining rural places in health policies and programs*. Iowa City, IA: Rural Policy Research Institute.

NCHS (National Center for Health Statistics). 2016. *Healthy People 2020 midcourse review*. Hyattsville, MD: National Center for Health Statistics.

NCHS. 2018. *Health, United States, 2017: With special feature on mortality*. Hyattsville, MD: National Center for Health Statistics.

NCHWA (National Center for Health Workforce Analysis). 2010. *Distribution of U.S. health care providers residing in rural and urban areas*. Rockville, MD: National Center for Health Workforce Analysis.

Possemato, K., E. M. Johnson, G. P. Beehler, R. L. Shepardson, P. King, C. L. Vair, J. S. Funderburk, S. A. Maisto, and L. O. Wray. 2018. Patient outcomes associated with primary care behavioral health services: A systematic review. *General Hospital Psychiatry* 53:1–11.

Probst, J., J. M. Eberth, and E. Crouch. 2019. Structural urbanism contributes to poorer health outcomes for rural America. *Health Affairs (Millwood)* 38(12):1976–1984.

Probst, J. C., W. E. Zahnd, P. Hung, J. M. Eberth, E. L. Crouch, and M. A. Merrell. 2020. Rural-urban mortality disparities: Variations across causes of death and race/ethnicity, 2013–2017. *American Journal of Public Health* 110:1325–1327. https://doi.org/10.2105/AJPH.2020.305703.

Pullmann, M. D., S. VanHooser, C. Hoffman, and C. A. Heflinger. 2010. Barriers to and supports of family participation in a rural system of care for children with serious emotional problems. *Community Mental Health Journal* 46(3):211–220.

Rhoades, E., and M. H. Derre Smith. 1996. Health care of Oklahoma Indians. *Journal of the Oklahoma State Medical Association* 89(5):165–172.

Rubin, R. 2020. COVID-19's crushing effects on medical practices, some of which might not survive. *JAMA* 324(4):321–323.

Rutledge, S. A., S. Masalovich, R. J. Blacher, and M. M. Saunders. 2017. Diabetes self-management education programs in nonmetropolitan counties—United States, 2016. *Morbidity and Mortality Weekly Report Surveillance Summary* 66(10):1–6.

Sandel, M., M. Hansen, R. Kahn, E. Lawton, E. Paul, V. Parker, S. Morton, and B. Zuckerman. 2010. Medical-legal partnerships: Transforming primary care by addressing the legal needs of vulnerable populations. *Health Affairs (Millwood)* 29(9):1697–1705.

Singh, G. K., and M. Siahpush. 2014. Widening rural-urban disparities in all-cause mortality and mortality from major causes of death in the USA, 1969–2009. *Journal of Urban Health* 91(2):272–292.

Spencer, J. C., S. B. Wheeler, J. S. Rotter, and G. M. Holmes. 2018. Decomposing mortality disparities in urban and rural U.S. counties. *Health Services Research* 53(6):4310–4331.

Talih, M., and D. Huang. 2016. *Measuring progress toward target attainment and the elimination of health disparities in Healthy People 2020.* Healthy People Statistical Notes No. 27. Hyattsville, MD: National Center for Health Statistics.

Thomas, S. R., G. H. Pink, and K. L. Reiter. 2019. *Geographic variation in the 2019 risk of financial distress among rural hospitals.* Chapel Hill, NC: North Carolina Rural Health Research Program, University of North Carolina at Chapel Hill.

van Dis, J. 2002. Where we live: Health care in rural vs urban America. *JAMA* 287(1):108.

Vest, J. R., L. E. Harris, D. P. Haut, P. K. Halverson, and N. Menachemi. 2018. Indianapolis provider's use of wraparound services associated with reduced hospitalizations and emergency department visits. *Health Affairs (Millwood)* 37(10):1555–1561.

Warne, D., and L. B. Frizzell. 2014. American Indian health policy: Historical trends and contemporary issues. *American Journal of Public Health* 104(Suppl 3):S263–S267.

Wright, B., E. Fraher, M. G. Holder, J. Akiyama, and B. Toomey. 2021. Will community health centers survive COVID-19? *Journal of Rural Health* 37(1):235–238.

Yaemsiri, S., J. M. Alfier, E. Moy, L. M. Rossen, B. Bastian, J. Bolin, A. O. Ferdinand, T. Callaghan, and M. Heron. 2019. Healthy People 2020: Rural areas lag in achieving targets for major causes of death. *Health Affairs (Millwood)* 38(12):2027–2031.